Heat Training Natural Hair 101

The comprehensive heat training guide for chemical free hair straightening and length retention.

How to use heat the proper way.

Loosening your curl pattern is possible without the use of chemicals.

Saleemah Cartwright, RN BSN

Entrepreneur, Registered Nurse, Licensed Cosmetologist, Author and Philanthropist. She is the Co-Founder and CEO of Healthy Hair Journey Enterprises LLC and the Hydratherma Naturals Healthy Hair Care Product Collection.

PREFACE

Let's Normalize Heat Training.

"UNPOPULAR OPINION- Heat is not the devil. The improper use of heat is. Remember that heat training natural hair is an option for you. I stand by heat training as a great alternative for those who are interested in chemical free hair straightening.

I absolutely love the heat training process. With heat training, the bonds of the hair are gradually loosened as time passes. It's great if you are thinking about becoming a "straight natural" or if you are thinking of relaxing your hair but would rather stay away from chemicals.
Right now, my hair blow dries pretty straight so I don't have to use much

heat when straightening with my flat iron. I can go out in the Atlanta humidity and it doesn't revert. I'm not wearing my natural curls right now so it doesn't bother me for my bonds to be loosened. I'm retaining length and my hair is strong and breakage free."

Saleemah Cartwright- Author

Does this scenario describe you?

So, you absolutely loveeee your natural hair. You have been wearing your curls for many years. Rocking your afro, twist-outs, braid-outs, bantu knot-outs and wash and gos have been so much fun. Also, protective styling has been a lifesaver when you don't feel like doing your hair and you want to give your hair a break from styling. It has been a really adventurous hair journey but something has been on your mind for quite a while now. You want to wear your hair straight. You have been trying to resist these thoughts because some judgmental members of the "natural hair nazis" are making you feel awkward or guilty about your thoughts of changing your hair. For a while now, you have been contemplating this change but you feel like you can't go through with it because you won't be true to your natural roots (by not wearing your hair in its curly virgin/natural state). You want to wear your hair straight for multiple reasons (which has absolutely nothing to do with not loving your curls). The main reason (on the top of your list) is TIME. Your hair is getting longer/thicker and your wash days are taking a big chunk of time out of your life. You are finding that it is taking 3-6 hours (or longer) to wash, deep condition, style and dry your hair. Since starting your natural hair journey, there have been many life changes that have occurred. Having children, starting a new career, dealing with aging parents and many other life changes have been sucking up a lot of your time. You just want an easier way to maintain your hair so that you can attend to these other areas of your life.

Now you are contemplating getting a relaxer to just make your life easier. Wash days will take only a few hours max and you will still look great without spending so much time on your hair. The hesitation to relax your hair comes from all of the possible health risks that are associated with hair relaxers. These health risks include multiple cancers, fibroids, hormone disruptions, Alzheimer's disease, cysts, reproductive damage, allergies and many other health-related issues. Because of these known health risks, you decided against relaxing and thought about keratin treatments because these treatments may be healthier. After doing extensive research on keratin treatments, you came to find out that these treatments release formaldehyde which is cancer causing as well. You found that there are many "formaldehyde free" keratin treatments containing the chemicals glyoxylic acid or glyoxoloyl carbocysteine but later found out that these treatments are not much safer because glyoxylic acid and glyoxoloyl carbocysteine actually both release formaldehyde when heated. You realized that the "formaldehyde free" labeling is very misleading and decided to ditch the whole keratin treatment idea.

You want your wash days to be faster and simpler. You want to keep your hair natural/chemical free and you want to wear your hair straight. What is the best option for you?

If this scenario somewhat describes you, I would suggest that you strongly consider heat training your hair.

In this book, I will share my story because the term "heat training" has such a negative connotation attached to it. When many hear the term, they automatically relate it to extreme hair damage, thinning, breakage and hair loss. I have to respectfully disagree with the heat training critics because if heat training is done properly, your hair will thrive for sure. This book will help those who are on a parallel path. Heat training may be controversial to many but if done the right way, HEAT TRAINING WORKS.

Why did I write this book.

Although I am a licensed hair stylist and have been for the last 25 years, I know that some of my fellow cosmetologists may be a bit upset with me for writing this book. Some believe that this type of styling technique should be left to professionals. Believe it or not, many stylists are not knowledgeable on heat training natural hair and may consider heat trained hair "damaged hair that needs to be cut off". This is not always the case and I'll go into detail about this a little later in this book. I have always been a person who believed in educating and empowering women "**who desire to**

do their own hair". If you do not feel comfortable with heat training your hair yourself, that is perfectly fine. This book is for individuals who feel confident in learning the process. It's definitely not rocket science. Heat training just consist of loosening the bonds of your hair slowly over time and if you have the right tools, the right techniques and the right products, you can do this!

I decided to write this book to educate those who are interested in embarking on their personal heat training journey. I have always seen "HAIR" from the unique perspective of "Cosmetologist" and "Client". I am a licensed cosmetologist and I have also been a client. I see both viewpoints.
Even as a stylist, I have never wanted my clients to be dependent on me

100% for the health of their hair. I believe that it is very important for clients to be educated on how to maintain their own hair and not to be 100% dependent on another person for this essential need.

When it comes to chemical processes, I personally believe that it should be left to a licensed stylist who has expertise in that area (i.e., color, relaxer, curly perms, etc.).

I also wrote this book to dispel the fear of using heat. As mentioned previously, "Heat is not the devil". Don't be afraid of using heat because it can actually help you on your healthy hair growth journey by keeping your hair in a stretched/straight state. Keeping your hair straight or stretched will prevent single-strand knots and will help you to retain length easier. I will discuss this more in detail later.

Many individuals will charge thousands to teach you how to silk press your own hair but this is not necessary at all! Learning to properly heat train and/or silk press your own hair is not extremely difficult to understand and practice makes perfect.

In this book, I will educate you on how to PROPERLY use heat to GRADUALLY heat train your hair. It will not happen overnight and you don't want it to. It's all about learning the proper process and you will learn this detailed process in this book.

*You are reading this book because you are interested in taking your heat training journey into your own hands. Do you want to become part of the straight natural hair community and wear your hair straight the majority of the time? I'll show you how. Let's get started.

TABLE OF CONTENTS

My Heat Training Story

Loosening my curl pattern intentionally. "I lost my curl pattern and I don't care."

I lost my curls and I don't care. Ohhhhhh. I know that it sounds cringe-worthy to some but if you bought this guide, you know exactly where I'm going with this.

My story:

Some of you guys may be familiar with my many hair journeys all the way back to the early 2000's on the "Long Hair Care Forum". If you were a member of this forum, you know that I have had just about every hairstyle known to man. Relaxer, color/bleach, pixie, texturizer, braids, mohawk, body perms, locs, shaved bald, twa, afro and the list goes on and on.

1

After wearing my hair in a short "Teenie Weenie Afro" for quite some time, I decided to grow my hair out again. With the exception of my 2 sets of locs, I was wearing big hair for the most part. Twist-outs, braid-outs and afros, were my go-to styles. On this hair journey that I embarked on in 2021, I wanted something a bit different.

I combed out my 2nd set of locs in 2020 and eventually big chopped my bleached hair color. As I began growing my hair out, I wasn't 100% sure as to what to do with it this time around. I know that I did not want to cut it anymore. I desired super long hair so I decided to embark on my waist-length journey. I was growing tired of my twist-outs / braid-outs and I was itching for a change. For the next 6 months, I just left my hair in protective styles until I decided what was next.

I have been extremely busy with my duties as the Hydratherma Naturals hair product line CEO and spending a lot of time on my wash days was not what I wanted to do anymore. I have thick 4 a/b hair and I exercise 3-4 times a week. I also swim frequently so I needed to cleanse and deep condition my hair more often than I did in the past. Don't get me wrong...Doing my hair is very therapeutic for me but I needed an easier wash day routine as my hair was gaining inches. Because of my busy lifestyle, I decided that wearing my hair straight was the best route for me.

Since I knew that I wanted to wear my hair straight, the 3 options for me were 1. to get a relaxer/texturizer again, 2. Brazilian Keratin Treatment or 3. to heat train my hair. I wasn't interested in doing a Brazilian Keratin Treatment because I didn't want to use formaldehyde-based products. While doing further research, I realized that the "formaldehyde-free" keratin treatment options are just as dangerous. I narrowed down my options and considered the pros and cons of each possibility.

PROS and CONS of a
Relaxer/Texturizer vs Heat Training

Relaxer / Texturizer

PROs

- No Reversion in the summer heat / reduced frizz
- Easier wash days
- Less time with general daily maintenance
- Less knotting and tangles
- Less or no shrinkage
- Easier hairstyling in general
- Hair straightens with less heat

CONs

- The use of chemicals with unknown long-term consequences
- Irreversible damage to the hair if done improperly

- Scalp burns/irritation
- Hair can become limp with no body
- Less natural shine due to mineral deposits
- It is a bit more difficult to maintain healthy hair and to retain length with chemical use
- The cost of a professional stylist to properly maintain the relaxer
- Only last 6-8 weeks requiring ongoing upkeep and dependence on the relaxer
- You cannot wear natural curls again until it grows out
- Dry hair issues are more prevalent
- Less hair volume

Heat Training

PROs

- Resistance to humidity- Depending on the level of heat training
- Increased shine and body/bounce due to no chemical deposits
- Can be less damaging to the hair when compared to the use of relaxers/ texturizers
- Has the benefits of a relaxer without chemical use / healthier alternative
- Can be DYI if educated properly on the procedure
- Less single-strand knots leading to split ends/breakage
- Easier to retain length when compared to the use of

chemicals / Decreased breakage
- Easier detangling sessions due to a looser curl pattern
- Easier to manage because the hair remains a in stretched state (Less time needed for daily maintenance)
- The hair is less resistant to moisture retention due to increased porosity (easier to moisturize)
- Able to see length due to decreased shrinkage
- Hair straightens with less heat
- More volume and less of a flat look
- Healthier scalp due to no chemical use

CONs

- The process takes time and is not instant (if done properly)
- Weakens the internal proteins of the hair
- The process is irreversible in most cases. Can cause permanently straightened hair pieces
- Your hair may not be able to be worn in its natural "curly" state any longer because the curl pattern may be uneven. It is very unlikely that you will keep your original curl pattern. Most of the time, straight pieces will be evident. Where the loosening will occur along the strand is highly unpredictable.
- Severe damage/breakage may occur if done improperly

- Requires patience and commitment
- May require the use of regular henna treatments or bond rebuilders to strengthen the hair bonds
- Requires time and commitment to a healthy hair regime. There are no shortcuts. A healthy hair regimen/schedule for deep treatments weekly (or every other week) must be maintained.

I measured the PROs and CONs of each. After thinking about it for a few months, I decided that heat training my hair was going to be my newest hair journey. The main determining factor for me was the fact that I didn't want to use chemicals any longer and heat training was more practical for my day-to-day lifestyle. As a matter of fact, I think that heat training gives similar or better results when compared to a relaxer. I have been a straight natural for almost 2 years. I use heat on my hair (in the form of a blow dryer / flat iron or both) every 2 weeks and my hair is not experiencing breakage, thinning or excessive split ends. My hair is THRIVING!

I am able to wash, deep condition/steam, blow out and flat iron my hair in 1.5 to 2 hrs. I get all of the benefits of a relaxer without the chemicals and the possible damaging effects. You can as well. I also love the shine and bounce of heat trained hair. There is nothing like it. I will continue to stand by heat training as a great alternative for those who are interested in chemical-free hair straightening.

Ok… So, let's back up a bit.

So, what exactly is heat training natural hair?

Heat training involves the repeated use of "direct" heat (in the form of a blow drier, flat iron or both) to slowly loosen the protein bonds of natural hair (intentionally) for easier straightening and less reversion. This should be done gradually taking weeks or months. As time passes, the hair begins to easily respond to heat making straightening easier. Your curls will loosen while heat training and you can loosen your curl pattern to the level in which you feel comfortable. I have seen heat trained naturals range from having a loose curl pattern to no curl pattern at all while maintaining the integrity of their hair.

Your hair is made of keratin which is a fibrous protein. The hair strand is made of an actual chain of proteins that grows from the hair follicle in the scalp. The 3 parts of the strand consist of the cuticle (outer layer), cortex (middle layer) and medulla (inner layer).

The cuticle (outer layer) consists of sheets of proteins arranged like scales on a fish and protects the inner layers of the hair. The cortex contains the pigment of the hair (melanin) and gives the hair strength and elasticity. It also determines the hair texture. The medulla is the most fragile portion of the hair strand and it contains your personal DNA.

These 3 layers of the hair strand are held together by bonds that combine to create a matrix. There are 3 types of bonds that link the protein chains together. The hydrogen bonds (weaker bonds), salt bonds (weaker bonds) and the disulfide bonds (strongest bonds).

The hydrogen and salt bonds are the weaker bonds and can be broken down with water or PH levels above 5.5. This allows for the hair to change its shape when wet. The disulfide bonds are the strongest bonds within the keratin and these bonds give your hair its texture. They are not easily broken down and can only be rearranged with prolonged heat use or chemicals such as relaxers, texturizers, curly perms and color.

Hair structure, strong links and weak links

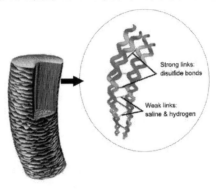

Strong links:
disulfide bonds

Weak links:
saline & hydrogen

When heat is applied to the hair
regularly, the keratin chains
rearrange themselves which loosens
the hair bonds. This occurs at temps
starting at 300 degrees F and above.
After the bonds are loosened, the
hair will remain straight or a looser
curl pattern will appear after the hair
is washed. Heat trained hair can still
be healthy hair without any breakage
occurring. The only change is the hair
no longer reverts to its natural curl

pattern because the bonds are permanently loosened.

Heat trained hair can range from just a slight loosened curl pattern to totally straight hair in its wet state. This will depend on the frequency of the use of heat and the temperature of the hair tools. If you follow my process, you will be able to loosen the curl pattern to where you feel comfortable and then dial back on the heat. Although it can be difficult to perfectly predict the curl loosening outcome, you can loosen your curl pattern slowly as time progresses to avoid major surprises.

HEAT TRAINING PROS – A more in-depth look.

I briefly mentioned the pros of proper heat training above and now I'm going to explain in a bit more detail.

A person who is considered a "straight-haired natural" is someone who wears their hair straight the majority of the time and rarely wears their hair in its natural curly state. Individuals choose to be "straight haired naturals" for a variety of reasons. Some people just like the look of sleek hair. Others feel that dealing with their hair in its natural state is too time-consuming and some want to retain length easier without having to deal with single strand knots or long detangling sessions on wash day. Many individuals with heat trained hair state that their hair has never been healthier.

If heat training is done properly, it becomes even easier to retain length and prevent breakage. This is because the hair is always in its straight/stretched state. There is less tangling of the tightly coiled hair strands and less knotting (single strand knots) to deal with. Also, the natural sebum from the scalp can easily pass from the roots to the hair ends when the hair is in a straightened state. This will aid in keeping the hair moisturized and preventing breakage. When the hair is tightly coiled, the sebum has a more difficult time passing down the hair strand because of the twist and turns that it encounters. This can result in dry ends if the hair is not properly moisturized on a regular basis.

Another change that occurs in the hair with heat training is increased porosity. With increased porosity, the hair can absorb additional moisture from the use of your moisturizers and treatments. Porous hair is a lot easier to moisturize so issues with extremely dry hair will lessen.

Heat training is a great alternative for those who have been considering relaxing their hair. Can you have healthy relaxed hair? ABSOLUTELY! Many of our Hydratherma Naturals customers use a relaxer and have extremely healthy hair. Years ago, when I used a relaxer, my hair was super healthy and I was able to retain length. At this point in my life, I do not want to use harsh chemicals recurrently on my hair and scalp. There are many individuals (like myself) who are cautious about using chemicals in general. The skin is not impenetrable so toxins do enter the body through the skin. Skin absorption rates vary among different parts of the body but the scalp has the maximum absorption rate. Toxins on the scalp and forehead are absorbed 4 times more than on other body parts due to the concentration of hair follicles. This is something that should be considered if thinking of using a relaxer or even a keratin treatment. Heat training natural hair is a practical and worthwhile option for many.

Are you worried about your hair going POOF in the humidity? As your hair becomes heat trained, it becomes more resistant to humidity. This is especially true with the correct silk press procedures and the right products. In most cases, heat trained hair remains straight in humid weather. I have worn my hair straight in the hottest Hotlanta heat and experienced very minimal reversion and sometimes none at all. Depending on your level of heat training, reversion is minimal (if at all). As your hair becomes heat trained, it becomes resistant to humidity. Using products containing keratin and silicones will prevent your hair from absorbing the humidity in the air as well.

Another significant thing to know is that heat training is not an extremely difficult method to learn. You can do it yourself if you are taught the proper procedure. Don't be intimidated. Be sure to take your time and have patience through the process because the progression is not immediate. It unquestionably takes commitment. Once you are educated in the process, you will be empowered to do your own hair which will save time and money.

Another PRO that I stated previously was that heat trained natural hair characteristically displays increased shine and body/bounce compared to relaxed hair. Relaxers leave sodium (lye) or calcium (no-lye) deposits on the hair which can cause the hair to be a bit dull. Also, the chemicals break down the disulfide bonds so fast resulting in less and less body after each relaxer session.

I recognize that many of these heat training benefits may sound a bit unusual to some. This is because so many of us were taught (for years) to stay away from heat and that the use of heat is bad for the hair. Now we know that the proper use of heat can cause your hair to flourish.

Heat training progress pictures.
Texture - before and after

The start of my heat training journey
4a/b

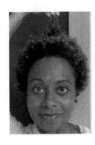 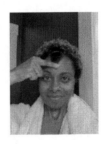

During my journey- The curl pattern is slowly loosening. I could have kept this curl pattern but I chose to loosen my curl pattern even more.

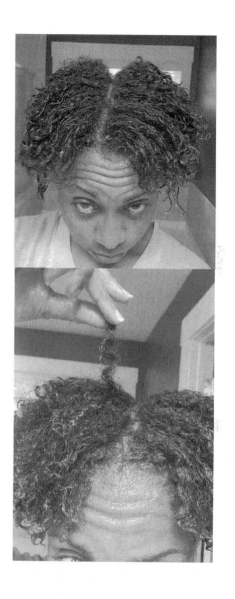

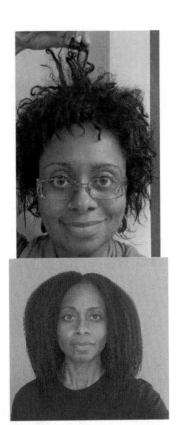

After further heat training. My hair in its wet state. The curl pattern is curlier at the root and straighter at the ends which is not abnormal for heat trained hair.

This is my hair blown out before flat ironing. My blowout is actually very straight now that I am heat trained.

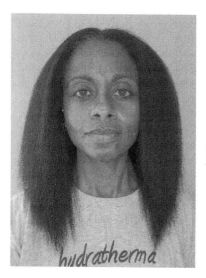

Flat ironing process using a ceramic iron and the Hydratherma Naturals Flat Iron Chase Comb.

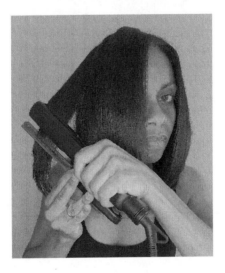

Completed silk press

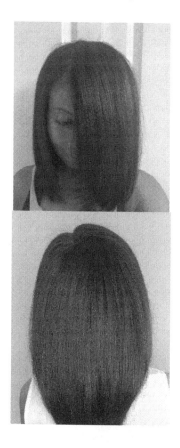

Retaining Length

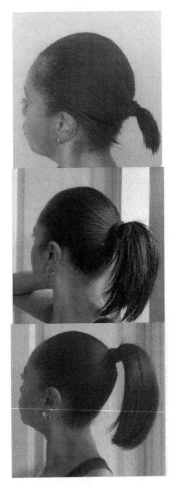

My Current Length

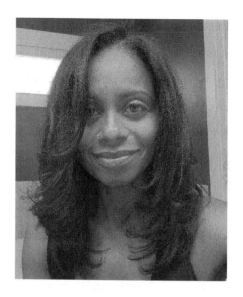

Is heat training for everyone?

Although heat training your own hair is a great alternative, it is not for everyone.

If your hair is currently in a damaged state, you wouldn't be a good candidate to heat train at this time.

It is extremely crucial to begin your heat training journey with healthy hair. Generally speaking, if your natural hair is strong and healthy, you should not have any complications with heat training (if the process is done properly). I wouldn't recommend heat training your hair if your hair is damaged and you are currently experiencing severe breakage, split ends or thinning. I suggest that you begin your healthy hair journey first and get your hair healthier over the course of 6 months to 1 year. During this time period, you will be cutting off your thin areas / split ends and staying consistent with your hair treatments. Transitioning out of your hair damage is crucial before starting your heat training journey.

I would also not suggest heat training your own hair if you have (lifted) color-treated hair or bleached hair. If your hair is currently colored (lighter) and you want to heat train your hair, I would suggest that you seek a professional stylist for heat applications and color maintenance. If not, it can be just too dangerous.

Heat training is for you if:

1. You love the look of straight hair and you do not want to use chemicals.

2. You have no problem being a "straight-haired natural" and wearing your hair straight daily.
3. You will be ok with running the risk of completely losing your natural curl pattern.
4. You want your hair to resist humidity.
5. You want easier washdays.
6. You want to retain length easier.
7. Detangling your hair feels like a grueling chore.

Heat training is NOT for you if:

1. You want to alternate between straight and natural curly looks.
2. You like to straighten your hair every once in a while.
3. You are afraid of losing your natural curl pattern.

4. You are apprehensive about the use of silicones.
5. You cannot invest in the proper hair tools and products.
6. You are impatient.
7. If your hair is damaged.

Before deciding to embark on your heat training journey, be sure to read through this book and weigh the pros and cons. Reflect on it for a while and then you will be able to make the right decision for YOU.

The Natural Hair Nazis

THERE IS NO "ONE WAY" TO WEAR NATURAL HAIR

Dear Natural Hair Nazis and the Hair Police. Please stop trying to police how others wear their hair. Black women have the right to do what we want with our hair. Natural, Relaxed, Curls, Straight, Weaved, Wigs, Braids, Heat-Trained, Afro, Locs, even the Jheri Curl is making a comeback.... whatever. Just ENJOY LIFE, BE HAPPY and DO YOU!

I know that heat training natural hair is a very controversial subject and many people just don't like the idea. Point blank... heat training bothers a lot of people and it is extremely troublesome to the Natural Hair Nazis.

Do you know who the Natural Hair Nazis are? They are individuals with 100% unprocessed hair who attempt to tell others what they can and cannot do with their hair. They are certain that it is their obligation to reprimand, harass and scold other individuals who choose not to wear their hair in its 100% natural state. They bash individuals who relax, color treat, wear extensions/wigs or who heat train. Oftentimes, they can be extremely judgmental and this causes needless division within the natural hair community.

The Natural Hair Nazis always question if someone is really "natural" if they straighten their hair. Wearing your hair straight is a rule violation to them. They believe that someone is "selling out" or not true to their African roots if they are not wearing their hair 100% natural all of the time.

Obviously, we know that his thought process is absolutely absurd but some individuals are bullied into wearing their hair in certain styles based on the opinion of others. Black women should do what we want with our hair without receiving backlash from others.

- If you decide that heat training is right for you, please don't listen to the Natural Hair Nazis. Tell them to have several seats. Be happy and confident with the decision that you have made on your heat training journey. It is your hair and it's your life.

- If you have been wearing your curly afro for many years and you decide that you want a change, IT'S ALL GOOD! I have changed my hair so many times and have experienced my share of criticism. Did it stop me from living my best life with my hair? NO WAY! Everyone will not support your decision but that's ok. One of the keys to happiness in life is doing what is right for you. Another key to happiness is minding one's business and that is what the Natural Hair Nazis need to do.

Heat Training vs Heat Damage

Is your hair still considered "NATURAL" if you heat train it?

Many individuals continue to argue about this meaningless dispute. I find these types of discussions extremely comical. I guess the answer to this question depends on who is being asked. If you ask me, I would say YES. I believe that heat trained hair is still natural hair as long as there are no chemicals being used. In my opinion, chemical-free hair is natural hair no matter how it is styled. If you ask the Natural Hair Nazis, I'm sure that the answer will be a resounding NO!

There is so much labeling going on in the natural hair community and life is too short for all of the judgement. "JUST LIVE" and forget about the labels. Wear your hair exactly how you want to and just enjoy your life.

The term "heat damage" can be debatable and divisive when used incorrectly. The prevention of severe damage is crucial to healthy heat trained hair. If the hair is severely damaged with the improper use of heat, it is generally irreparable. The best way to treat severely heat-damaged hair is to avoid hair damage in the first place. This book is here to help you do just that.

So, does heat trained hair = heat damaged hair? Lots of individuals routinely associate heat trained hair with the term "heat damage". Because of this, there are countless individuals who are deathly afraid of using any type of heating tool (even a hooded dryer). Although the bonds of the hair are permanently loosened with the constant use of heat, the hair can still be very healthy, breakage free and length can easily be retained.

If you want to be "EXTREMELY TECHNICAL", heat training is a mild, slow and tremendously controlled form of "heat damage" because the hair is no longer in its virgin/natural/untouched state. The natural curl pattern is not 100% intact but this does not necessarily signify damage. If heat training is done properly, the bonds of the hair are loosened but not to the point where breakage, splitting and thinning will occur. The term "damage" is very subjective. In my opinion, severe heat damage occurs when the bonds of the hair are "totally destroyed" causing breakage, loss of elasticity, no shine, thinning, dryness and excessive split ends. The hair can be extremely stiff and does not style well. This characteristically happens when heat is overused/used improperly. This situation can unquestionably be avoided with the proper application of heat. The key is the fact that the bonds are being loosened on purpose and you are aware of the big picture.

If you look at the anatomy of the hair under the microscope, there are changes that occur during the heat training process. Yes... the curls are permanently transformed but the hair can still be healthy and thrive. In other words, the bonds can be broken causing a looser curl pattern without triggering massive breakage/damage. It is easy to move from heat training to severe heat damage if the process is not done correctly. Severe damage can be avoided with the right heat training practices.

I know that it sounds like a giant oxymoron. How can the hair be mildly damaged and be healthy at the same time? Heat trained hair can definitely FLOURISH and be extremely healthy. We do have many examples of this. I, myself is an example along with many other heat trained / natural haired youtubers such as the Glamtwinz. There are also numerous celebrities who have gorgeous heat trained natural hair such as Skai Jackson, Kenya Moore, Queen Latifah, Reginae Carter, Jordyn Woods, Cardi b, Oprah Winfrey, Kerry Washington, Kash Doll (who achieved her waist length goal with heat training) and the late Prince, Aaliyah and LongHairDontCare2011 from YouTube- RIP.

There is a fine line between severe heat damage and heat training.

Ok. We are going to be honest here. Can someone use heat incorrectly and cause severe hair breakage, split ends and hair injury? Absolutely! This is what I would unquestionably consider "severe heat damage".

Some may define heat damage as a slightly loosened curl pattern due to a change in the hair's bonds. That is absolutely fine as well but we have to remember that if the bonds are loosened, the hair can still be considered healthy. Healthy heat trained hair can be breakage free and can also retain length. Split ends, hair loss and extreme breakage do not have to occur if heat training is done properly. All in all, curl loosening can be considered good or bad depending on what you want. Since you are reading this book, you will most likely not be alarmed when you see that your curl pattern has changed. This is most likely one of your objectives on this journey.

The terms heat damaged and heat trained are used interchangeably a lot. The answer to the question of whether the hair is heat trained vs heat damaged will vary depending on whom you ask. If the loosening of the curl pattern was planned, it may be considered heat training by the willing participant. If it was not planned, it may be considered heat damage by the shocked client who wanted to keep her curls.

As long as your hair is healthy, loosening your curl pattern will only worry you if you want to go back and forth between curly and straight.

Scenarios:

EBONY

Ebony straightens her 4 a/b hair every 2-4 weeks (for the past year) and noticed a loosening of her curl pattern. She also sees some completely straightened pieces of hair mixed with her loose curls. There is no breakage evident and she keeps up with her hair trims every 3-4 months (resulting in negligible split ends). Her hair is getting longer as well... even with the scheduled trims.

NIA

Nia unquestionably loves the look of her 4 b/c curls and wore her hair in a huge afro regularly in the past. Lately, she has been wanting to wear her hair straight just for a change of pace. She decided to treat herself and has been frequenting a popular salon to let them give her silk presses. After each salon visit, she noticed that her hair was softer and her curls were just slightly more loosened. After her 4th visit to her stylist, her curl pattern was similar to a 3 b/c hair texture. She is not experiencing any breakage or split ends.

Ebony and Nia are both asked if they are experiencing "heat damage".

Ebony is a "straight-haired natural" (AKA a person with natural hair who predominantly wears their hair straight). She may consider her hair "heat trained". She may answer… "My curls are super loose and I have some straight pieces because my hair is heat trained. It doesn't bother me at all. My hair is growing out very well and I'm retaining length. My hair also doesn't revert in the humidity because my curls are looser and I absolutely love that. I don't mind that my curls are not the same when my hair is wet because I don't wear my natural curls anyway".

Nia (a person who loves to change things up), may have a different response. She may respond in this way… "On wash day, my curls were so loose and stringy, it's not breaking off but my curl pattern is entirely different. This is not what I was expecting. I want my beautiful tight curls back. My hair is totally heat damaged and I have to cut it off because I can't wear my hair in its natural state. I'll have to start over and grow out the "damaged" loose ends". My hair is completely damaged and I'm so angry that I allowed someone to use so much heat on my hair. I will never use heat on my hair again. This experience was the worst ever!"

As you can see, the answer to the "heat damage" question can be awfully subjective especially when there is no breakage, dryness or splitting occurring. The issue revolves around the fact that they both had different expectations. Who is right and who is wrong? In actuality, both answers can be accurate. It just depends on the perspective. Different perspective / same thing. The most important question is, what was the intention? Essentially, a loosened curl pattern may be considered "heat damage" if that wasn't the true intention from the beginning.

In my professional opinion, there is a spectrum of levels to which the bonds of the hair can be loosened. Heat trained hair is hair with very minimal heat damage. In other words, it is low on the spectrum of "damage". If the bonds of the hair are broken in any way, the hair is not in its 100% natural state. This doesn't necessarily mean that the hair is experiencing breakage and shedding. As mentioned previously, your hair can be both healthy and heat trained.

Healthy "Heat Trained" Hair Characteristics:

- **Good elasticity-** The hair's ability to "snap back" to its original state when stretched out.
- **Shine-** Resulting from an intact cuticle (lying flat) causing light to easily reflect off of the strand.
- **Smooth texture-** Never feeling dehydrated and brittle because the hair is easier to moisturize.

- **Minimal breakage-** Due to increased elasticity and the hair constantly being in its stretched state.
- **Normal shedding-** 50-100 strands per day is considered normal.
- **Negligeable split ends –** Supports length retention because split ends travel up the strand and ultimately break off.
- **Easy detangling –** The hair is softer and there is a lot less friction between hair strands.
- **Holds and responds well to moisture-** Also resulting in a healthy cuticle.
- **Has movement body and bounce-** Due to healthy elasticity.

- **Under the microscope-** Cuticle layers look smooth, tight and intact. Negligible split ends.

Damaged "Heat Trained" Hair Characteristics:

- **Overly dry and brittle in appearance-** Resulting from a damaged cuticle.
- **Severe breakage and thinner hair ends-** Typically, more hair is noticed in the comb (short hairs and longer strands as well).
- **Split Ends-** Due to lack of scheduled trims.
- **Decreased elasticity-** When the hair is stretched, it doesn't bounce back and usually breaks off immediately.
- **Dull dry appearance-** Light doesn't reflect off of the hair

easily because the cuticle is not lying flat along the hair strand.

- **Tangles galore-** The flat exterior of a closed healthy cuticle makes it easier to comb and brush through. When the cuticles are unhealthy and raised up, hairs easily tangle and tend to get caught on one another.
- **Stiff hair-** Lack of body due to decreased elasticity.
- **Feels rough-** An unhealthy cuticle and split ends will cause the hair to have a rough feeling.

A person can also evaluate hair damage by examining the hair strand under a microscope. Under the microscope, the cuticle layer of the hair strand is open, disordered and destroyed. You can also see small breaks along the strand. Numerous split ends are most likely evident as well. Healthy hair will have an intact/closed cuticle layer that appears smooth and homogeneous. Hair that is severely damaged will display raised and broken areas along the cuticle. With extreme damage, the hair is totally stripped of its cuticle layer.

 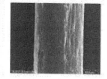

WEAK DAMAGE   MODERATE DAMAGE   HIGH DAMAGE

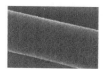 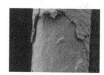

Healthy Cuticle Layer   Raised Cuticle Layer   Damaged Cuticle Layer Missing Scales

Length Retention While Heat Training.

Why Healthy Heat Trained Hair Retains Length.

Can you still use heat and retain length? ABSOLUTELY!

Many people are shocked to find out that you can actually retain length easier while heat training (if the process is done correctly with the correct methods, tools and treatments). The main reason why heat gets a bad rap is because it is being used incorrectly. As we all know, the incorrect use of heat will cause breakage on the hair ends and severe split ends. This will definitely impede length retention. I have been able to easily retain length with the regular use of heat. I typically use heat every 2 weeks. There are many other heat trained / "straight natural" individuals who are easily retaining length with the use of heat.

The reason why the proper use of heat (in the form of flat ironing and/or blow drying) aids in length retention is because these processes keep the hair is a stretched state. Hair in a stretched state is less prone to tangles because stretched hair strands are less likely to loop around its neighboring strand causing tangles. Your comb can easily glide through your hair without popping, snagging or breaking off (less manipulation). There will also be a decrease in single-strand knots which is a major cause of breakage.

As you progress on your heat training journey, you will notice that your hair will become a lot softer and easier to manipulate on wash days as well. This is because the bonds of your hair are loosening up with the use of heat and your hair will detangle easier. Easy detangling definitely contributes to less overall breakage. Detangling my heat trained hair is an absolute breeze.

Many women with natural waist-length hair have 1 major thing in common and that is the use of heat in the form of a blow dryer, flat iron or both. Some of them have been using heat for 20 years or longer. I had a great friend in college named Leah and she had a head full of thick natural waist-length hair. I had no clue what heat training was back then but I remember her telling me that she blow-dried and used the straightening comb on her hair after each wash. She did this for many years (since she was a child) and she never had a relaxer.

Yes! Heat trained hair can retain length.

What You Will Need

Ok. Now that you have the foundation, let's get into the good stuff!

What you'll need to have for the healthiest heat training journey EVER!

Exceptional Styling Tools.

Before you get started on your heat training journey, there is one thing that is nonnegotiable. You unquestionably have to invest in 5-star styling tools. This doesn't mean the "most expensive" styling tools. I have a few great recommendations for you that are comparable to the popular/expensive brands. Just keep in mind that you will have to make an investment in the proper hair tools in order to have a successful heat training journey. We absolutely cannot cut corners here.

Hair Dryer

All hair dryers are not created equal.

One of your first investments will be in a salon-quality hair dryer. The blowout process is one of the most critical steps in the heat training method and it is the foundation of your heat training journey. I will explain why later in this book. The blow dryer will help to determine the sleekness of your silk press so investing in a good one is extremely important. There are many advancements being made in hair-drying technology. This can make choosing a hairdryer overwhelming for some but I will make the choice much easier for you.

Since you have decided to embark on this heat training journey, you absolutely want a sleek professional looking blowout. I would certainly recommend a Nano Tourmaline / Ceramic Blow Dryer. These types of dryers are specifically coated inside with ceramic / tourmaline. The ceramic portion provides even heat distribution along with infrared heat. The tourmaline (a rare gemstone) coating also produces infrared heat with negative ions.

These types of blow dryers dry the hair from the "inside to the outside" of the hair strand (due to infrared heat technology) which allows for faster drying time. A faster drying time is definitely what you need in order to help mitigate severe damage. Unlike traditional dryers, ceramic/tourmaline dryers dry the hair up to 50% faster because of the even heat distribution (no hot spots along the shaft). It takes me about 15 minutes to blow-dry my arm pit length hair. With ceramic / tourmaline technology, the hair is dried evenly and negative ions are produced. These negative ions do not open the hair shaft. It actually locks in moisture by sealing the hair cuticle, repelling humidity and reducing frizz. The right blow dryer will give you smooth and sleek results before even using the flat iron.

All blow dryers labeled ionic are not necessarily high quality. I do not suggest purchasing a blow dryer that is only labeled "ionic". This is because "ionic dryers" do not provide the ceramic/tourmaline technology for even heat distribution. If the hair dryer is labeled ceramic/ tourmaline, it also produces negative ions. The ceramic/tourmaline combo is the absolute best choice.

*Sleek comb attachment- I also suggest purchasing a comb attachment if your dryer doesn't come with one. If you are a beginner when it comes to getting a smooth blowout, this will make your life a lot easier.

*Price Range- $100.00 and up

Ceramic / tourmaline hairdryers are slightly more expensive than traditional ionic hairdryers but the added benefits make them worthwhile

Flat Irons

Ceramic vs Titanium Flat Irons for Heat Training

Ceramic or Titanium flat irons. Which one should you choose? This really depends on your hair type, the speed in which you would like to heat train your hair and the results that you want to achieve. There is a big difference between ceramic and titanium flat irons. The differences are evident in how quickly the plates heat up, durability and what method they use to allocate heat to your hair. Have you ever noticed that the final outcome of your silk press doesn't look smooth, shiny and straight? This may be occurring because of the plates that are being used. Be sure that the plates are fully (ceramic or titanium) plates and not just coated ones. Higher-quality flat irons are made with full ceramic/titanium plates. Let's break this down.

Ceramic flat irons are irons with ceramic plates. These irons do not heat as fast as titanium irons do. As with ceramic hair dryers, ceramic flat irons heat the hair from the inside to the outside of the hair strand and provide even / gentle heat distribution (without hot spots). This type of iron has a lower chance of burning your hair because it doesn't reach higher temperatures when compared to a titanium flat iron. "Not getting as hot" can be considered good and/or bad. This just depends on your hair because ceramic irons may require more passes. Heating the hair from the inside to the outside would be considered "gentler" when compared to the titanium iron which heats up the surface of the hair shaft. Because of this, ceramic flat irons are commonly considered a safer selection. This is especially true for someone with thin or fine hair. Ceramic irons also produce negative ions to prevent frizz and the iron easily glides through the hair without tugging. This can result in less damage from snags. Ceramic irons are not as durable as titanium irons so they may not last as long.

Titanium irons are irons made with titanium plates. The titanium iron is the newest technological advancement for styling tools. For myself, it is my favorite and I personally use titanium irons on my medium-textured hair most of the time. It distributes heat from the surface of the hair only. It also produces negative ions to seal the cuticle (preventing frizz). This gives more smooth and shiny results. This type of iron is extremely durable and it heats very quickly. Titanium irons are popular among professional stylists because they transfer heat fast. Titanium irons get very hot and can cause damage faster if used improperly. Because the iron gets extremely hot, fewer passes are necessary. Slightly lower temperatures are advised for beginners as well. If you use a titanium iron, your hair will be smooth, silky, glossy and polished for days or even weeks.

So which iron is better for you?

This will depend on your hair texture and density. (Fine, Medium or Thick)

For thin, low-density and fine hair, I recommend starting with a ceramic iron. Fine hair is the most fragile of all hair textures and it is prone to severe damage (if heat training is done improperly). If your hair is very soft and easy to straighten, a ceramic iron would be your best bet.

For medium to thick textures, hair that is coarse, kinky / tightly curled or more tolerant to heat, I recommend a titanium iron to heat train your hair. If your hair is very thick or coarse, a ceramic iron may not be strong enough to heat train your hair. Ceramic irons may also require additional time to achieve the heat training results that you'll quickly receive with a titanium iron.

If you would like to progress very slowly on your heat training journey, I would suggest starting with a high-quality (fully plated) ceramic flat iron. As I mentioned previously, be sure to stay away from the "coated" irons. Using a high-quality ceramic iron will loosen your curls very slowly. The ceramic flat iron is great for those who are just testing the waters with heat training because it is less aggressive when it comes to straightening the hair. If you don't want to jump in the water head first, definitely start with ceramic technology. Just keep in mind that using a ceramic iron to heat train will require a bit more patience if your hair texture is medium to thick or if you have a course hair type that is difficult to straighten. Using ceramic technology may take twice the length of time to heat train when compared to using a titanium iron. You can always start with a ceramic iron and switch to a titanium iron later if your needs change.

If you want to be a bit more aggressive with your heat training journey you can start with a titanium flat iron on a slightly lower temperature setting. Titanium Flat irons will straighten your hair more aggressively. I started my heat training journey with titanium irons and I do not regret it at all. My hair is 4a/b medium textured. Those with kinkier coils or hair that's harder to straighten will definitely benefit from using titanium plates to heat train.

*Tip- Some flat irons do not allow for exact temperature settings adjustments in degrees. The settings may only display "high- medium-low". I suggest that you stay away from these types of irons. It's extremely important to find a flat iron with adjustable heat settings so that you can safely adjust the temperature (up or down) slowly to the exact degree that you want.

An extremely general rule of thumb. If you have medium to thick hair, you can commonly go "UP TO" 450 degrees F max. If you have thin, fine hair, you should stay under 400 degrees F. I will go into much more detail about temperature settings later. Some flat irons heat up to 470 degrees. I do not suggest setting your flat iron to temperatures above 450 degrees (even on extremely coarse / thick hair) because this can result in scorching of the hair.

If you are starting with a ceramic iron and feel as though your hair is not progressing fast enough on your heat training journey, you can alternate every other heat treatment with ceramic and titanium technology. In other words, you can buy both irons and alternate these irons with each flat iron session.

*Honorable mention- Tourmaline flat irons for normal/medium to coarse hair.

I am not a huge fan of tourmaline flat irons because these irons do not produce long-lasting results based on my experience using them. I believe that they do deserve an honorable mention because they also produce negative ions which can be beneficial for most hair types. If you are looking for a moderately gentle iron but you are indifferent when it comes to long-lasting results, you may want to try the tourmaline iron. It actually produces more negative ions than ceramic irons. This is because tourmaline is often infused into ceramic and titanium plates.

Flat Iron Sizes

The length and thickness of your hair is the determining factor when it comes to the size flat iron that you purchase. The right size iron will allow you to straighten your hair more efficiently and decrease the risk of severe hair damage.

If your hair is shorter, I would recommend 1-1.5 inch plates so that you can straighten smaller sections.

For longer / thicker hair, 2-inch plates will work just fine. This way, you can cover more surface area.

If you are still unsure which size to purchase, I would recommend a 1.5-inch plate flat iron because it can be used on long or short hair. You can also get closer to the root areas a lot easier when compared to the 2-inch plates.

There is also the pencil flat iron. The pencil flat iron has super narrow plates (3/10 inch) for hard-to-reach areas in the nape, roots and the edges. You can use the rat-tail comb to comb your edges forward, then use the pencil flat iron to straighten them. The pencil iron is great to have but not a necessity.

*Price range for any excellent quality flat irons- $40.00 and up.

Steamers

When it comes to your heat training journey, steaming is an absolute must. Steaming is the process of using moist heat / humid water vapor to restore moisture by hydrating the hair. Hair that is exposed to heat on a regular basis is prone to extreme dryness. Because of this, steaming clearly benefits heat trained hair. Steaming opens the hair cuticles so deep conditioning treatments can be better absorbed. You can even use less conditioner and get the same results because of an increase in product absorption. The steaming process also increases the hair's elasticity, prevents brittleness and softens the hair strands. This ultimately leads to reduced breakage. The health of your scalp also benefits from the use of steaming. It detoxes the scalp and increases collagen production as well. It provides heat and hydration to the scalp which stimulates blood flow. Increased blood flow to the scalp also contributes to rapid hair growth.

While heat training, I prefer the benefits of steaming when compared to covering the hair with a plastic cap and sitting under a hood dryer. Although the hood dryer deep conditioning method works well, your hair will hydrate much easier with the steaming process.

~Hair Tips:
-Always use a deep conditioning treatment on your hair before

steaming for ideal moisture retention.

-Don't cover your hair with a plastic cap while steaming because this will prevent the ultimate absorption of your deep conditioning treatments.

-Don't steam longer than 20 minutes. This may result in "over moisturizing" of the hair. Over moisturizing can make your hair too soft resulting in breakage. 10-20 minutes of steaming is enough to hydrate your hair properly.

Price range: There are many different professional hair steamers on the market ranging from $60.00 and up. Since steam is steam, you can opt for a hand-held clothing steamer. This is what I use on my hair and it works just as well as the expensive steamers.

- Professional Hair Steamer- $60.00 and up

- Hand-held clothing steamer- $15.00 and up

*Hot Combs- Hot combs seem to be making a small comeback but I often wonder if it is a good or bad thing. There are some technologically advanced hot combs out there using ceramic and titanium plug-in technology. These serve as an alternative for those who feel more comfortable using them. You can definitely heat train your hair using a hot comb. If you decide to go this route, I would recommend staying away from the old-school hot combs that you place directly on the fire or portable stove. It is very hard to regulate the temperature and also the old-school hot combs don't utilize ceramic / titanium technology. They can be very damaging to the hair's cuticle layer.

All in all, when it comes to silk pressing natural hair, I have noticed that hot combs don't give the smooth/shiny results that I love. They can also snag the hair and cause breakage as time passes. I'm not a hot comb advocate so I won't be discussing them much in this book. In my opinion, the flat iron is the superior choice when it comes to heat training.

Additional Tools Needed

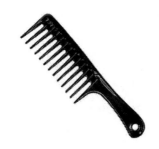

Wide Tooth Comb- High-quality wide tooth comb for detangling your hair. As you heat train your hair and your hair grows out, you will notice that your roots / new growth will be kinkier than the rest of your hair. This comb will really prove to be beneficial for detangling the roots and your hair ends.

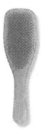

Detangler Brush- High-quality detangling brush for detangling and distributing products through the hair.

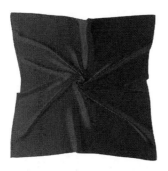

Opened Bottom Loc Sock, Turban or Silk/ Satin Scarf- For securing your wrapped hair while sleeping / silk press maintenance.

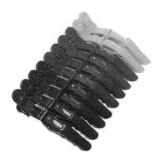

Clips – For sectioning the hair during the heat training process.

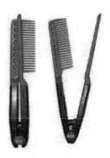

Flat Iron Chase Comb- For a smooth press from root to tip without frizzy ends.

Available at
www.HydrathermaNaturals.com

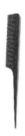

Rat Tail Comb – For parting ½ inch
sections during the flat ironing
process. Also, great for parting your
wet hair before applying your silk
press products.

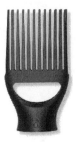

Comb Attachment for Blow Dryer-
Helps to attain a smoother blowout.
Works amazingly well for beginners
and for those with experience.

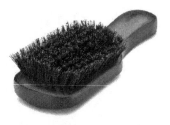

Boar Bristle Brush- This particular
brush is one of my personal favorites

because it works amazingly well to smooth your edges after flat ironing your hair. It also works great for smooth / pulled back hairstyles such as ponytails and buns. The fibers of these brushes are made to distribute your hair's natural scalp oils more evenly from the roots of your hair to the ends while easily getting rid of shed hairs. This distribution of oils will make your hair super shiny. This brush is a must have. Just be sure that the bristles are not too firm.

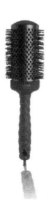

Round Brush- This brush can be used with a blow-dryer to help obtain a smoother blow out. This is not recommended for beginners but I wanted to add this brush as an alternative for those who feel confident enough to use it. It can cause hair elasticity problem if used regularly. This brush should only be used occasionally on afro textured hair. If you do not want to use this brush, the blow-dryer comb attachment works just as well and it's less damaging.

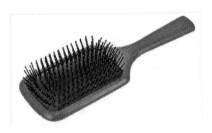

Paddle Brush- This particular brush is great for wrapping your hair at night. It can also be used during the blow-drying process for those who are more experienced.

Silk Press / Heat Training Professional Hair Care Product List

Using the wrong products on your hair can cause your heat training journey to be a very unsuccessful one. It can result in the burning of your hair after just one application of heat. Using the right products to protect and increase the elasticity of your hair is extremely vital. You have to make an investment in excellent / salon-quality hair care products to have a successful heat training journey. You can't use "run-of-the-mill" products and expect exceptional results.

Clarifying Shampoo- Clarify. Never flat iron hair that is not properly cleaned. A sulfate-based deep cleansing shampoo is very important when it comes to heat training. There is so much controversy about the use of sulfates but SLS is the absolute best cleansing agent. Nothing in the market cleanses the hair like it. It is extremely essential to deep cleanse your hair prior to the silk press process. If your hair is not properly cleansed, extreme damage can occur (and fast) because excess residue/buildup will be baked into your hair. This causes extreme dryness and breakage right away. Also, a clean slate is necessary so that your deep conditioning treatments can easily enter the strand during the steaming process. Hair that is clean will result in a silk press that is shiny, bouncy and damage free.

Moisturizing Shampoo- After deep cleansing the excess dirt/product build from your hair, add moisture to your hair with the use of a moisturizing shampoo. You can use this type of shampoo for your second lather to increase your hydration levels. This can be a sulfate-based shampoo or a sulfate-free moisturizing cleanser. Avoid shampoos that are very oily.

Deep Conditioning Treatments- These treatments are extremely necessary to keep your hair strong and should be done with a steamer for the best results. It is so important to keep your hair balanced with moisture and protein because too much of either can cause breakage. A great regimen will include alternating a light protein treatment with a moisturizing treatment every other week to allow your hair to fall into a nice balance of protein and moisture. When heat training, you can also add a few additional protein treatments as needed without worrying about protein overload. If you have previously considered yourself to be protein sensitive, please don't be too concerned about this issue while heat training. Heat trained hair tends to be more porous so a bit more protein can be used to fill in the porous gaps. This will add strength. If you have decided to incorporate henna with your regimen, you will need to deep condition with protein a lot less because henna acts as a protein treatment although it is not one.

Leave-In Conditioners / Heat Protectant- For added protection against hair damage, a leave-in conditioner containing silicone and light proteins (such as vegetable proteins / keratin) is needed. Some people are deeply anxious when it comes to using silicones. This is an unwarranted fear. If you are heat training your hair, silicone will become your bestie. When heat is being used, silicones add an extra layer of protection so that your hair will not burn. It helps to remove tangles easily making the hair a lot more manageable during the heat training preparation process. Silicone will also prevent/minimize reversion by protecting the hair from humidity. Silicone and any other product residue will easily be removed during your weekly clarifying/cleansing sessions. Be sure that your leave-in heat protectant is very lightweight, smooth in texture and not sticky.

There are many types of silicones including dimethicone, cyclomethicone, cyclopentasiloxane, amodimethicone, dimethicone, dimethiconol, phenyl trimethicone, and dimethicone copolymer to name a few. Using a deep conditioner containing some type of silicone is enormously advantageous while heat training. Dimethicone is the heaviest type of silicone. This particular type of silicone will give your hair a brilliant shine and incredible slip before your press. It provides a great barrier to heat.

Serum- Heat Protectants- Serums add an additional layer of protection and a brilliant shine. An excellent salon-quality serum will contain silicone and keratin. Keratin is one of the most important proteins found in your hair naturally and it plays an important role in forming a protective layer on your hair. Keratin will protect your hair from humidity, fills in cracked cuticles, adds strength to your hair shaft, eliminates frizz and adds shine. A great serum will allow your flat iron to easily glide through your hair without causing snags.

*No Oils- Do not use oils for heat protection. Oils heat up very fast and can result in immediate burning of your hair. The oil will literally "fry" your hair. Many people underestimate how damaging this can be.

Hair Bond Rebuilders -There are a few hair bond rebuilding products in the market that may help you on your journey. Bond rebuilders claim to work at a molecular level to help restore broken disulfide bonds. I personally don't use them but I am not averse to using them at all. Many people swear by the use of bond rebuilders and I would recommend them as opposed to not using anything to strengthen your hair while on your heat training journey. Bond rebuilders are not my favorite because they will provide only a temporary fix to your hair. These products require many steps and only work with frequent applications. Because of this, multiple steps have to be taken when applying the products during each wash day. They are made of synthetic ingredients and can be extremely costly. Bond rebuilders may be a good option for those who have bleached or high-lift hair colors to strengthen however, there are cheaper protein-based treatments that work just as well.

Henna -When compared to bond rebuilders, I believe that a healthier alternative is the use of all-natural henna.

Henna is an all-natural plant that is native to northern Africa. Also known as Lawsonia Inermis. It comes in a powdered form. It has been used on the hair and skin for over 5000 years. Henna binds to and strengthens your hair shaft permanently so it is not just a temporary fix. The important component that contributes to its strengthening properties is the molecule tannin. Tannin binds to the keratin fibers permanently. It does this by winding around the actual keratin fibers, making the strands physically stronger.

Although henna is not a protein treatment or a bond rebuilder, it acts as both (but permanently). It fills in any porous gaps along your hair strand. This builds the cuticle and protects the cortex layer which proves to be tremendously helpful during the heat training process. Henna gives the hair an incredible shine and actually makes each hair strand thicker, softer and smoother.

Henna contains the compound lawsone which has staining properties. Lawsone also binds to the keratin protein in the hair giving the hair a rich reddish color. Hair stylists tend to dislike henna because it can be difficult to bleach or apply hair color over it. This is because Henna is permanent. Also, many hairstylists find that the application processing time is too time consuming (henna needs to sit on the hair for 1-4 hours).

Henna Pros

- It is 100% natural.

-Henna strengthens the hair permanently. The permanent binding/coating of your hair cuticle will prevent severe heat damage/burning of your hair.

- Makes the hair smoother.

– It is not necessary to apply on each wash day.

- Henna can be used as often as you like without causing damage. I apply henna to my hair every 2-3 months with great results.

-It's cheap! Henna is incredibly inexpensive and can be purchased on Amazon or at your local Indian grocery store.

-While heat training, henna will also soften your curls and slightly loosen your curl pattern even more because each actual hair strand will weigh more. This is due to the plant deposits along the cuticle. This can be a pro or a con but I have this listed as a pro because it can speed up your heat training (curl loosening) process without causing damage and without changing the chemical structure of your hair.

– It will actually make your hair thicker because each hair strand is coated.

-It prevents reversion when your hair is exposed to extreme humidity. This is because the henna particles bind to the porous gaps along the hair strand. This prevents the hair from absorbing much of the humidity in the air.

Cons:

-Henna is not for those who like to experiment with hair colors because you cannot use commercial dyes on top of henna without possibly causing damage.

-Your roots will need to be processed as your hair grows out. You may reapply henna to your hair ends for strength and to add a more vibrant reddish color without any issues.

-Long application times. Henna should be processed for 1 hour minimum.

- All henna treatments MUST be followed with an intense moisturizing steam treatment (using a hydrating deep moisturizing conditioning treatment) because henna can be very drying. If not, breakage can occur.

-Henna gives the hair a reddish tone and this may be a pro or a con depending on your preference.

~Henna Hair Tips:

- If you decide to try henna, be sure that the henna that you purchase is 100% pure and not mixed with metallic dyes. Read the ingredient list before purchasing because some products labeled as "henna" contain many chemicals.
- I apply henna to my hair from root to tip every 2-3 months. As mentioned previously, you can apply henna as often as you like. It is not necessary to apply more than once a month.
- Always follow your henna treatments with a hydrating/moisturizing deep conditioning treatment. Henna is not a protein treatment but it acts as one so your hair will need to be hydrated after using it.

- You may add conditioners, coconut milk and oils to your henna mixture for added moisture while processing.
- If you have a stylist, it is very important to let your stylist know that you are using henna in your hair. This is especially true if you are looking to color your hair.

*Honorable Mention

Dry Shampoo- During the latter days of your silk press (leading to wash day), you may notice that your hair lacks body and that it appears a bit oily. This typically happens at the 2-week mark. This is due to the natural oils being secreted from your scalp and from any products that you may have added to your hair during the week. Dry shampoo can be used to absorb any excess oils from your hair. It will easily collect the oils that may have built up on the hair and scalp. This will make the hair look less greasy. It will also keep the hair cool/dry and increase volume/body. Great for people who work out and sweat a lot at the gym. There are many oil-free / dry shampoos in the market. Honestly, they all basically work the same so avoid the more expensive brands. In general, dry shampoos are great for absorbing oil and odors.

The Detailed Silk Press Process

Start to Finish

Straightening natural hair has definitely come a long way since the "hot comb on the stove" days. That was indeed a form of heat training however, if you had someone do your hair who wasn't experienced with controlling the heat of the hot comb, your hair can be burned immediately on contact.

25 years ago (when I was in cosmetology school), I had a traumatic hair experience happen to my client and I. I remember flat ironing a client's hair with the marcel flat irons at my beauty school. I was very inexperienced and didn't know how to maintain a certain temperature with the irons. My Caucasian instructor

wasn't too knowledgeable about how to use these types of irons either. I ended up leaving the marcel flat irons in the oven for longer than I should have. When I applied the flat irons to my client's hair, it immediately burned her hair off (from the root) on contact. We all just heard a sizzling sound and the whole room smelled like burnt hair. A section of her hair was burned off and fell to the floor. It was extremely upsetting for both of us. Thankfully, the breakage was at her nape area so we could cover it up. She agreed to receive free hair treatments on a weekly basis. I would never forget that learning experience and since that day, I became very conscious of how to use heat the proper way.

There are many steps that need to be taken to receive a beautiful silk press. If you skip over certain steps, your silk press results can be stiff and dull looking. In this portion of the book, I will guide you step by step on what to do to obtain the best silk press with bounce, shine and body!

The Cleansing Process

The best silk press results start at the shampoo bowl. Some of you may have heard this term. The cleansing process is one of the most important steps in obtaining the best silk press on your heat training journey. If your hair is not properly cleansed, you will be actually baking dirt/build-up into the hair while using your heat tools. This can result in severe dryness, damage, breakage and hair loss as time passes (or immediately). It is very important that the hair be properly cleansed so that your deep conditioning treatments can be easily absorbed.

As mentioned previously, 2 shampoos are necessary. A deep cleansing clarifying shampoo needs to be used for the first lather to remove any dirt and buildup from your hair/scalp. If there is a lot of buildup on your hair, you may have to repeat this process until your hair is cleansed properly. You can then follow up with a moisturizing shampoo for the 2nd lather. This will add moisture and hydration to your hair. Be sure that your hair is rinsed extremely well and that all of the shampoo is removed.

*Beneficial Hair Cleansing Tips

- To avoid hair tangling, braid your hair into 4 big braids prior to shampooing your hair.
- Make sure that your scalp is properly cleansed as well. If you have a lot of buildup on your hair and scalp, apply the clarifying shampoo directly to your scalp and hair before wetting your hair. Massage the shampoo into your hair (focusing on the scalp) then wet your hair and scalp. You can exfoliate your scalp using a toothbrush, shampoo brush or just with the tips of your fingers. This will give you a great cleanse on the first lather. This exfoliation process will increase blood circulation

to the follicles and will promote hair growth as well. A clean scalp will help prevent shedding because excess sebum can clog the hair follicles and cause inflammation.

The Deep Conditioning Process

The conditioning process is another crucial step that will determine how well your hair responds to heat training.

After rinsing the shampoo from your hair, apply your hydrating deep conditioning treatment to your hair from root to tip. At this time, I suggest that you section your hair into 4 sections and comb through your hair with a wide tooth comb (while saturated with deep conditioner). Then follow up with a detangling brush to ensure that all of the tangles are removed.

Now is the time to steam your hair with your steamer. As mentioned previously, direct steaming is preferred during the heat training process and should be done with each heat training session. Using direct steam really makes a huge difference when it comes to hydrating the hair and retaining moisture. I suggest steaming the hair for 10 to 15 minutes. I like to use my hand-held clothing steamer. I typically part my hair in 2 sections and cover one section with a plastic cap. To the uncovered section, I steam for 10 minutes. Then I switch sides. Make sure that your hair stays very moist during the steaming process. You can spray water on your hair while steaming if necessary. There is no need to steam for longer than 20 minutes. This can result in over-moisturizing the hair. Over-moisturizing the hair will cause the strands to become too soft and can result in breakage.

Here are a few benefits of hair steaming:

- Allows for deeper penetration/absorption of moisture, vitamins and minerals to each hair strand. This will ultimately strengthen your hair.

- Increases elasticity which leads to easier manageability.

- Less breakage and easier detangling occur because your hair is properly hydrated.

- Increases shine and improves the appearance of your hair.

- Gives the hair a soft, smooth, brilliant, radiant and silky look.

After steaming, rinse your hair thoroughly. The last 10 seconds should be a cold rinse. This will help to close the cuticle. When the cuticle is closed, moisture is locked in and the hair will have a healthy shine. Make sure that all of the deep conditioner is thoroughly rinsed from your hair. Be sure not to leave any residue. This is very important because you don't want to use heat on hair that has lingering products in it. This will cause burning.

Correctly Preparing the Hair for The Use of Heat

Using the proper products prior to the use of heat is vital on your heat training journey. Using a protective leave-in conditioner AND serum (containing silicones and keratin) will prevent your hair from burning. It is important to use both (leave-in conditioner and serum) for an added layer of protection while heat training.

After rinsing out your deep conditioner, your hair should be fairly detangled. Section your hair into 4 sections with your rat tail comb. To each section apply a pea-sized amount (shorter length hair) to a dime-sized amount (longer length hair) of your protective leave-in conditioner and follow up with a pea to dime sized amount of your protective serum. Always start with the smallest amount of product to prevent your hair from being weighed down. Comb through with a wide tooth comb and follow up with your detangling brush. Using the brush is very important at this stage for even distribution of the products throughout your hair.

*Hair Tips

-Be sure that your hair remains wet while applying the protective products. Use a spray bottle if necessary and place hair in bantu knots to hold in the moisture.

-Don't overuse the heat protective products. Just a little is all that you need. Adding too much leave-in conditioner and serum will weigh down your hair.

The Blow-Drying Process

Using the proper blow-drying technique will contribute to the smoothness of your silk press. It is important to have a smooth blowout prior to flat ironing your hair. Your blowout will determine how many passes you will need to do with your flat iron. A smooth blow-out will result in using fewer passes with your flat iron. All in all, the key to an amazing silk press is in getting your hair as smooth as possible while blow-drying. As you heat train, you will notice that your hair will blow out straighter (and faster) with ease.

If your hair is naturally kinky (my hair is- 4a/b), you will notice that your hair will blow dry into an afro when you initially start on your heat training journey. As your heat training journey progresses, you will notice that your blowout will become straighter (from roots to ends) and less heat will be necessary. The way that your hair responds to heat will change as the disulfide bonds in your hair release. Less heat will be necessary for a long-lasting straight look and less reversion will occur.

After applying your protective products brush your hair sections to evenly distribute the products. Proceed to blow dry each section until completely dry on a medium to high heat setting.

*Hair Tips

- To ensure that you obtain the smoothest blowout, I suggest utilizing a high-quality comb attachment for your blow dryer. This is especially true if you have less experience with blowouts because it will make blowing your hair out a lot easier. The comb attachment is my favorite tool to use for a smooth blowout. If you are a bit more experienced when it comes to blow drying your hair smooth, a paddle brush can be used while blow drying your hair as well.

- I do not recommend the long-term use of round brushes while blow-drying your hair. Round brushes can weaken the elasticity of your hair with the constant stretching of the hair strands. Weakened elasticity of the hair can definitely cause long-term problems on your heat training journey. Round brushes should only be used occasionally on afro textured hair.

- While on your heat training journey. I absolutely do not suggest air drying your hair prior to flat ironing. Not using a blow dryer before flat ironing will require you to use more direct heat with your flat iron (resulting in more passes). Air drying can cause more tangling and single-strand knots as well. Studies have shown that abusing a blow dryer can cause damage to the surface of the cuticle but air-dried hair displays more damage to its cortex which is more troublesome. Damage to the cortex is very difficult to manage and more difficult to recover from.

The Flat Ironing Process

As you proceed on your heat training journey, flat ironing your hair will become a piece of cake! If your hair was straightened appropriately during your blow-out process, your flat ironing session should be a breeze.

As mentioned previously, choosing a high-quality flat iron is very important if you decide to heat train your hair. A great ceramic or titanium iron will slowly release your hair bonds if used correctly.

REVIEW- So, let's discuss heat temperature settings again. If your hair is fine/thin, I recommend keeping your temperature setting under 400 degrees F (350-400 degrees F). There is no need to go much higher with this hair type.

For medium to thick/coarse hair, 400 to 450 degrees F is appropriate. Under no circumstances should you exceed 450 degrees because this will cause scorching of the hair. The above-listed temperature settings for fine/medium/thick hair are general guidelines. When choosing the right temperature setting for your own hair, be sure to keep in mind how your hair has responded to heat in the past.

Section your blow-dried hair into 4 or more sections and take very small/thin sections of hair. Flat iron each section from root to tip. Taking very small/thin sections (roughly ½ inch thick) is very important to ensure even heat distribution and a smooth press from root to end. I do not suggest passing the iron over each section more than 3 times. If you notice that there is steam coming from the iron during the flat ironing process, don't be alarmed. If you used heat-protectant products, you do not have to be concerned with your hair burning unless the temperature is above 450 degrees F. Heat-protectant products will create steam when coming in contact with direct heat.

To add more body to your silk press, you can lower the temperature of your flat iron and create curls. You can leave the curls in or wrap your hair after curling.

During the first few months of your heat training journey, you may notice that your hair may not be "silky straight" on the first try (unless you use an extreme amount of heat) and this is absolutely normal. You may also notice that your hair may revert faster in humidity. This is normal as well. Hair that is not heat trained normally reacts this way. The longer you heat train your hair, you will notice that your silk press will become progressively smoother and increasingly resistant to humidity. This heat training process takes patience. As your disulfide bonds loosen, your hair will respond to heat differently. As time passes, less heat will be necessary to straighten.

*Hair Tip

-To get a smoother press from root to tip, I recommend the "Chase Method". The chase method involves the process of running a fine or moderate tooth comb or brush through your hair simultaneously along with a flat iron. Placing a rat tail comb or a specialized chase comb in front of the flat iron stretches the hair and will provide tension while using heat.

Product recommendation: The Hydratherma Naturals Flat Iron Chase Comb. Unlike a rat tail comb or a brush, this comb will actually grip the hair providing more tension. This results in a smoother press from root to tip without the frizzy ends.

As you can see, the perfect silk press doesn't depend on buying the most expensive flat iron. It starts with the cleansing process, deep conditioning products/methods (steaming), along with the blow-drying process. All of the prep-work prior to the actual flat ironing process is very important.

As I mentioned previously, "Heat is not the enemy, it is the improper use of heat that is". Using heat responsibly is crucial while heat training. You will have a very successful heat training journey if you follow these extremely valuable steps. Always remember that any process can be modified during YOUR journey based on the results that YOU want to receive.

5 Additional Recommendations for a Successful Heat Training Journey

1) Know your hair texture.

Knowing your hair texture is very important when starting your heat training journey. This will determine how much heat your hair can take without burning. Hair textures consist of fine, medium and thick hair. You can determine your hair texture by using a piece of thread. If your hair is thinner than the thread, your hair would be considered fine. If it is the same diameter, it would be considered medium. If your hair has a larger diameter than the thread, it is thick or coarse. It is not necessary to use very high heat settings with fine hair.

2) Know your hair's history with heat.

Heat training natural hair is not a one size fits all regimen. Before you actually get started on your heat training journey, consider how your hair has responded to heat in the past. What heat settings have you used previously and how did your hair respond to certain temperatures? Did your hair previously respond better to ceramic or titanium irons? Have you experienced hair burning in the past or severe damage? What caused it? You may or may not be able to answer most of these questions adequately however, knowing how your hair has responded to heat in the past will help you set your baseline when starting your heat training journey.

3) **Decide what heat tools you will be using on your heat training journey.**

Whether you use a blow dryer, flat iron or both for heat training is really up to you. You can heat train your hair with the use of a blow dryer alone. The results will take longer because it is a less aggressive approach to heat training. It is an option for those who just want to test the waters when it comes to loosening the bonds of their hair. With the blow dryer-only technique, your hair will progressively become softer as time passes. You will also notice that your drying time will decrease and less heat will be necessary for smoother blow-outs. Your blow-outs will become less "bushy" as time progresses. Just keep in mind that heat training with only the use of a blow dryer will require patience. It will take much longer but it is a great option for those who really want to take their time on their heat training journey. It is a great option for those who don't like the silky straight look but still desire to heat train for easier wash days. The "blow dry only" heat training technique is also great for those who want to maintain most of their curl pattern.

If you do love the silky straight look and you want to progress a bit faster on your heat training journey, I recommend using a blow dryer and flat iron. The heat training journey is still a process that takes time however, it will take a reduced time period to heat train if you go this route. Decide if you want to proceed with a ceramic or titanium flat iron for your journey. Maybe you would like to alternate the irons with each heat training session. Be sure to review the "Ceramic vs Titanium Flat Irons for Heat Training" section of this book to decide which iron is best for you based on your hair's thickness/type/ texture.

All in all, use the heat training tool(s) that you feel comfortable with. You can always change things up as you proceed on your journey based on the results that you are achieving.

4) Start with a lower heat setting and work your way up.

Whether you start with a ceramic or a titanium iron, I absolutely recommend that you start off with a lower heat setting and work your way up (if necessary). This is the best way to avoid burning your hair. Even if your hair is thick and coarse, I don't suggest starting with a heat setting of 450 right away. Everyone's hair reacts to heat differently so keeping track of the heat settings that you use (with each heat training session) is so important. If your hair is fine or highly porous, I would recommend starting your heat training journey on a temperature setting of 350 degrees F and increasing the heat settings by 10 degrees F with each session until you notice a noticeable change in the softness of your hair. For Medium to thick/low porosity hair, I suggest starting at 400-420 degrees F and working your way up with each heat training session. If you notice a beneficial difference in your hair while using lower temperature ranges, there is no need to increase your heat settings.

5) **Create a heat training schedule and a journal reporting how your hair is responding to heat.**

Creating a schedule and sticking with it is very imperative. There is no race to the finish line when it comes to heat training your hair so take your time to avoid setbacks. You should decide when you will be using heat on your hair each month. This can be a weekly, every other week or a monthly heat training schedule. During these heat training sessions, you can decide between blow drying alone or blow drying (and flat ironing) your hair. Be sure to write down how your hair responded to each session and evaluate what you want to do next.

Casual Heat Training Examples

Example 1- "I will heat train my hair with a blow dryer monthly to see how my hair responds and then increase my heat sessions to include blow drying 2 times a month based on how my hair responds to heat." This method would be for those who what to proceed with extreme caution. If you have extremely fine and highly porous hair, this method might be right for you. Heat training your hair this way will keep your hair in a stretched state and will not include any direct heat with the use of a flat iron so the heat training process will take a bit longer.

Example 2- "I will heat train my hair every 2 weeks. I will use only a blow dryer on week 2 and blow dryer with a titanium flat iron (on "X" temperature setting) on week 4. This is a great technique for those with medium to thick hair who desire a medium / aggressive approach.

Example 3 – "I will heat train my hair every 2 weeks with a blow dryer and flat iron. I will use a ceramic flat iron on the first session of the month and a titanium iron for the second session." This method is recommended for only those with medium to thick hair. Be sure to monitor your hair closely. This is the method that I currently use on my hair.

Example 4- "I will heat train my hair every week with a blow dryer and ceramic or titanium flat iron on X temperature setting." This is a more aggressive method and is recommended on thicker / coarse textures while closely monitoring your hair. If you have a medium hair texture and you know that your hair tolerates heat well, you may be able to start your journey this way also. My hair is medium textured and I used this method for the first few months of my heat training journey. I then decreased my heat training sessions to every two weeks which is what my current regimen is.

As you can see, there are many alternatives that you can take. I recommend starting off with a less aggressive approach and working your way up. This does not mean that you ABSOLUTELY have to start with the least aggressive approach. Just make your decision based on your own comfort level, your hair's history with heat and your hair's texture/type/condition and porosity.

Take things month by month. At the end of each month, describe how well your hair responded to your heat training sessions in your journal. At this point, you can decide how to proceed for the next month. Ask these questions. Has my hair's porosity changed? How is my hair's elasticity? Does my hair feel much softer? Have my curls loosened? Do I feel comfortable with the curl pattern that I currently have? If you are happy with the current condition of your hair, proceed with your same routine or you can lower the temperature settings on your tools a bit. There is no need to become more aggressive if you are happy with your hair at this point. If you would like to see more of an increase in the softness of your hair, a looser curl pattern and a longer-lasting silk press, you will need to become a bit more aggressive the next month. This can be done by increasing the heat settings by 5-10 degrees, switching from a ceramic to a titanium iron or increasing the frequency of your sessions. If you feel like your hair is progressing too fast, you can always take a break from heat training (i.e., skip a month), lower the frequency of your heat training sessions or decrease the temperature settings on your styling tools.

In your journal be sure to document heat settings, hair porosity changes, hair softness, hair elasticity, tools used and frequency of sessions per month.

Monitor Your Hair Closely

Monitor your hair closely after each heat training session.

Be sure to monitor your hair thoroughly and pay close attention to your hair's porosity and elasticity.

Hair Porosity Changes

Hair porosity is defined as a measurement of the hair's ability to absorb and retain moisture. It can also define how easily moisture can penetrate each hair strand. Low porosity hair doesn't readily absorb moisture or treatments. High porosity hair absorbs moisture easily but is unable to retain it. Hair porosity is mainly determined by genetics, but the use of heat and chemicals can increase the hair's porosity.

The use of heat will certainly increase porosity levels in the hair. As the bonds are being broken, the hair becomes more porous and small gaps may be evident along the cuticle layer. This is why treating your hair with protein treatments and/or henna treatments is so important. These types of treatments will fill in the porous gaps along the hair strand and will strengthen your hair. The use of silicones will also help to temporarily seal the porous gaps.

Steaming is extremely important for low and high-porosity hair. It will increase the absorption of moisture in low-porosity hair and will aid in moisture retention for highly porous hair.

As mentioned previously, highly porous hair cannot tolerate very high heat settings. You can observe your hair's porosity by taking a strand of your shed hair and putting in into a glass of water. If the strand sinks slowly to the bottom of the glass, your hair has normal porosity levels. If it quickly sinks to the bottom, you have high porosity hair. If it doesn't sink at all and floats on top of the water, you have low-porosity hair.

As you heat train you may notice that your hair is becoming more porous as time passes. This is fine as long as you keep up with your hair protein/henna treatments, steam treatments and use your heat-protectant products containing silicone.

If you notice that your hair is more porous than you are comfortable with, you can take a break for a few weeks and treat your hair with protein and/or henna. Because henna will permanently lower the porosity levels of your hair ends and will fill in any porous gaps, you can resume

your heat training sessions
immediately after using it.

Hair elasticity changes.

Hair elasticity is defined as how long
a single strand of hair can stretch
before returning to its normal state.
You can test your hair elasticity by
taking a strand of shed wet hair. Hold
the strand at the ends and gently
stretch the strand. If your hair
stretches and bounces back, your hair
has great elasticity. If your hair strand
doesn't fall back into shape or if it
breaks, your hair elasticity is low.

As you heat train, it is very important
to monitor your hair elasticity. You
may notice a slight decrease in your
hair elasticity as you progress on your
heat training journey and this is
normal. You do not want to lose all of
your hair elasticity because this will
result in breakage.

After each heat training session, monitor your hair elasticity. If you are noticing that your hair elasticity is decreasing, you can increase your elasticity by hydrating your hair properly. Balancing the moisture and protein levels in your hair will prove to be very beneficial in maintaining healthy hair elasticity. This can be done with the use of moisturizing steam treatments, daily moisturizing products, protein treatments and/or henna treatments.

Hair changes that you will notice as time passes- overview

As you proceed on your heat training journey, you will detect many noticeable changes in your hair. The first thing that you will notice is that your hair will become softer when in its wet and dry state. Your hair will be a lot easier to manipulate and detangle on your wash days. Your hair will also feel less coarse (while wet and dry). This is because of the loosening of the disulfide bonds.

It will take less time to style your hair and less heat will be necessary. You will experience faster blow-drying sessions and your blowouts will be straighter and smoother. It actually takes my hair just under 10 minutes to blow dry. Your hair will straighten easier and you will only need one pass with your flat iron on your hair ends. You will also notice that a lower temperature setting will be required to straighten your hair with your flat iron.

As you heat train, another positive change that you will notice is that your hair will be more resistant to reverting in humidity and your silk press will last a lot longer. As the disulfide bonds loosen, your hair is less likely to revert in even the hottest temperatures. I will discuss why this occurs later in this book.

You will ultimately see less breakage because your hair is in its stretched state the majority of the time which makes it easier to manipulate. The number of single-strand knots evident will decrease considerably. Eventually, all of your single-strand knots will be completely cut off if you keep up with your regular trim schedule.

Curl loosening will be apparent at varying degrees. The level of curl loosening is difficult to predict however, as time passes, your curls will definitely elongate (especially if you are using henna treatments). While heat training, it is incredibly difficult to maintain your virgin curl pattern and most heat trained naturals could care less about keeping their virgin curl pattern because they are not wearing their hair curly anyway. The longer you heat train, the more your curls will loosen. When your hair is wet, you will notice that your older hair (hair ends) will have a looser curl pattern (or none at all) and the hair closer to your roots will have a tighter curl pattern. Please don't panic if you notice that your hair ends are straighter. This is completely normal while heat training. Your hair ends will be straighter because they have been exposed to more heat. When your hair is in its straightened state, this is not at all noticeable.

All of these noticeable changes will contribute to faster and easier washdays. All in all, my wash day takes roughly 1.5 hours (on average) from start to finish and this includes cleansing, my 20-minute relaxing steaming session, blow drying and flat ironing. I take my sweet time but if I'm in a time crunch, I can get it done faster. On days when I blow dry only, it will take much less time as well.

How Long Will It Take to Heat Train My Hair.

This really depends. There are many factors to consider.

- Your hair type/texture – Fine/thin/porous hair will heat train faster than medium/thick/coarse hair.

- The type of flat iron that you use. Titanium flat irons will heat train more aggressively when compared to ceramic irons.

- The frequency of your heat training sessions. Of course, weekly heat training sessions will progress faster than monthly sessions.

- The degree to which you would like to have your curls loosened (which is a personal preference). Do you want just a slight release of your curl pattern or something more dramatic?

A slight release will take just a few heat training sessions. I have seen some heat trained naturals go from 4a/b to 1c straight hair and everything in between (from loose curls to waves). Heat training to obtain looser curl patterns or straight hair will take longer. I wouldn't recommend loosening the curl pattern to completely straight because it isn't necessary to receive the benefits of heat training.

That being said, heat training can take anywhere from a few months to a year depending on how aggressive you are. The important thing to remember is that you can always make adjustments as you proceed on your journey. I.e., "increase or decrease" the temperatures of your styling tools or "increase or decrease" the frequency of your heat training sessions.

The Maintenance of Your Heat Trained Hair

You have reached your desired level of curl loosening. What do you do on silk press day?

Has your hair already softened to your liking? Did your curls loosen to your desired state? Is your silk press lasting a lot longer in the humidity? If you are happy with where you are on your heat training journey at this time, it is all about maintaining your hair's strength and integrity. You can approach your silk press day less aggressively now that you have reached your heat training goal. Here are a few tips.

Reassess your temperature settings- Now that you are where you want to be on your heat training journey, you can lower your temperature settings on your flat iron. There is no need to use a higher heat setting because at this point, your hair straightens very easily. When I first started my heat training journey, I started out with a heat setting of 450 degrees F. Now that my hair is properly heat trained, I maintain my hair with a heat setting of 430 degrees F and I may use an even lower temperature setting in the future. If I want more of a textured press and not a silky straight look, I use a heat setting of 400 degrees F.

Heat training the roots only- Don't be afraid to "tap those roots" in order to maintain your heat trained hair. As your hair grows out, focus on the roots with your flat iron. During your silk press sessions, you can do a few passes on the roots to blend with the smooth ends. I recommend 2-5 passes on the roots and one pass on the hair ends. This method will loosen the bonds of the roots as they grow out. Your hair roots have a tighter curl pattern and can handle a few more passes to blend with your heat trained hair. I typically maintain my heat trained hair with around 5 passes on my roots and one pass on my hair ends.

Switch flat irons based on your preferences- If you have been heat training strictly with a titanium iron, you may now consider strictly using a ceramic iron if you wish. Now that your hair is heat trained, less heat is necessary and ceramic irons are less harsh on the hair. A titanium iron may not be necessary for you at this point but this for your you to judge. You can also alternate between the use of a ceramic and titanium irons with each silk press session. I personally like to alternate my flat irons because I love the look of my hair after using a titanium iron.

Take breaks if you want to- Now that your hair is heat trained, you can definitely take breaks if you feel that you want to. You can sometimes wear your hair in protective styles for 3–4-week timespans being sure to keep up with your cleansing and conditioning schedule. You can blow dry your hair and braid it up in cornrows. My go-to protective styles are wigs or headwraps. When I remove my protective style, it is always fun to see how much my hair has grown when I straighten it again. These days, I haven't been protective styling much because my hair has been doing very well without the use of protective styles. Just know that it is definitely okay to take breaks.

Be very consistent with your cleansing and deep conditioning schedule- To maintain healthy heat trained hair, it is critical to maintain a consistent cleansing and deep conditioning schedule to keep your hair hydrated. It is very important to steam your hair with each deep conditioning treatment for maximum moisture retention. This can be done weekly or every 2 weeks. I don't recommend extending your washdays longer than 14 days because your heat trained hair needs extreme moisture. Your hair cannot absorb moisture (optimally) in a dirty state. Prioritizing your steaming treatments will help increase elasticity and hydration levels. Both are extremely important with heat trained hair. Hydration is crucial for a smooth blowout and will help the cuticle to lay flat.

Be consistent with your protein and/or henna treatments- I mentioned the importance of protein and henna treatments previously. These treatments are needed to fill in the porous gaps along the hair strand and this strengthens the cuticle layer. If you decide to incorporate henna into your hair regimen, I recommend performing henna treatments every 2-3 months. Although henna is not a protein treatment, it acts as one. If you are doing henna treatments on your hair, you do not need to perform protein treatments frequently because henna performs the same as protein would. If you are not using henna, you can use light protein treatments on your hair every 2-4 weeks. Light protein treatments are better for your hair when compared to heavy protein treatments. Heavy protein treatments can be very harsh and can sometimes cause protein overload.

Maintain the moisture and protein balance in your hair- Those who are familiar with me are fully aware of the fact that I am a firm believer in balancing the moisture and protein levels in the hair. My husband and I created a product line based on this crucial balance of moisture and protein called Hydratherma Naturals products. I wanted to create products to maintain this moisture/protein balance with a simple regimen. Too much protein can make your hair hard and cause breakage. Too much moisture can cause the hair to be too soft (over moisturized) which can also lead to breakage. How do you know which one your hair needs? The best time to determine if the hair is balanced is while the hair is wet. After washing and deep conditioning your hair, look at one hair that has shed. Lightly tug the strand of hair. If your hair is spongy or gummy when it is wet, more protein is needed. If (when wet) it breaks right away when you pull (without much elasticity) you need more moisture. Listen to your hair and it will definitely tell you what it needs. If you want to get more information on balancing the moisture and protein levels in your hair, take a look at our website www.HydrathermaNaturals.com On our site, we go into much more detail about the process and what products to use. In short, be sure to balance the use of your moisturizing and protein deep conditioning treatments. You can alternate your protein and moisturizing treatments after each cleansing session and eventually your hair will fall info a great balance of moisture and protein. Once your hair is balanced, your hair will become healthier. You will notice a lot less breakage and even more length retention.

Only apply heat to your hair on your wash day - **No exceptions.** Heat free styling in between heat training sessions is a must. Your hair should always be in an ultra-clean state before using heat. If you are using heat on hair that is not clean, you will burn your hair immediately or progressively as time passes. Even using lower temperature settings is not actually safe. Any product buildup or natural oils (sebum from the scalp) will heat up rapidly and this is what actually causes the burning of the hair. To avoid this, try heat-free styling to add curls to your hair. For example, bantu knots, pin curls, soft rollers, flexi rods or steam curls-molecular rollers.

Keep up with your hair trimming schedule- Trimming your hair is absolutely necessary while heat training. Using heat can increase the occurrence of split ends because of the way heat affects the cuticle layer of the strand. If you have severe split ends, start with a "haircut" to get rid of ALL of your split ends. This may hurt your soul at first but if this isn't done, you will not be able to achieve your healthy hair goals and your heat training journey will not be successful. After cutting off all of your split ends, resume your trimming schedule. You will be astonished at how well your hair retains length. Split ends will continue to travel up the hair shaft (causing breakage) so it is so very important to cut them off and prevent them from coming back with frequent trims. I suggest trimming your hair every 3-4 months while heat training for general maintenance. I trim my hair every 4 months and my hair is thriving.

Don't overuse heavy products-
Adding too many heavy oils/creams is not necessary on your heat training journey. Here is a great tip and this is what I do. During the first week of my silk press, I add very little product. I typically only add the Hydratherma Naturals Herbal Gloss Heat Protector to my hair for extreme shine and UV ray protection. During the 2nd week (leading to wash day), I'll add my moisture and protein-balancing products to my hair. I use only a pea-sized amount of each of the Hydratherma Naturals Protein Balance Leave-In Conditioner (adds protein), Daily Moisturizing Growth Lotion (adds moisture) and the Hair Growth Oil (to promote growth and

to seal in the moisture). During this time (week 2), I play around with styles such as heatless curls, buns or ponytails.

Have a simple nightly routine- I suggest that you keep it simple with your nightly routine. On most nights, I wrap my hair. I think that it is the best way to keep your silk press looking sleek and it also eliminates the need to bump your hair with heat the next day. If you are not sure how to wrap your hair, there are plenty of online videos demonstrating this. We also have a hair wrapping tutorial on our www.HealthyHairJourney.com website. If opting for curls, try pin curls or soft rollers. Remember to not "overuse" oils and creams to avoid product accumulation. Just a pea-sized amount is all that you need per application. Also, reduce friction and breakage while you sleep with the use of silk/satin scarves or loc socks. If you are not interested in wrapping your hair, try a long du-rag to keep your hair in place at night. Parting your hair down the middle and using the crisscross method (crossing the hair in the back) with a satin bonnet is great as well. This is especially true if your hair is extremely long.

Workout / exercise tips to maintain your silk press- Keeping your silk press looking great can be challenging if you work out and sweat a lot. There are some things that you can do to keep your hair looking as fresh as possible. I work out 3-4 times a week and I manage to keep my hair looking extremely nice during the week. What works really well is keeping your roots stretched during your workout. After your workout is complete, the key is letting your stretched roots completely dry before styling. A great example would be wearing your hair in two ponytails. Two ponytails are better than one because more air can get to the middle of your scalp. With just one ponytail, you'll tend to get more reversion at the root area (especially in the middle of your head). After the hair is completely dry, you can proceed to wrap your hair and let it set for a smoother finish. If you don't have much time, you can also use a cool dryer only on your roots (while wearing the ponytails and before wrapping your hair) for faster drying time.

Showering tip- Maintaining your silk press in the shower is quite simple. Be sure that your hair is wrapped securely with your silk scarf. You can add an additional silk scarf for added protection. Cover your hair with a plastic cap. Then, place a headband around the outside base of the plastic cap to block out water and excess humidity. The headband serves as a seal to better protect your hair from swelling. I call this the double-wrap method.

Always have a raincoat and/or umbrella nearby- Now that you are a straight natural, be sure to keep hooded raincoats and umbrellas handy just in case. The reusable/plastic hooded raincoat is small enough to carry in your purse just in case you unexpectantly need it.

Maintain your general health- As you heat train your hair, it is important to remember that healthy hair is also a reflection of what is going on inside of your body. Maintaining a healthy lifestyle and being sure to take in important vitamins and minerals are very important. Taking care of yourself will help to ensure healthy hair growth and will help to minimalize shedding. Eating well, exercising, drinking plenty of water and taking hair supplements (if necessary) are all helpful.

As you can see, heat trained hair is "low maintenance" but not "no maintenance". Daily styling is going to be much easier for you however, being sure to keep up with your steaming /hydration treatments, trims, etc. is of vital importance.

Don't Do This. Learn From My Mistake.

I made this blunder on my heat training journey.

Here is the key mistake that you should absolutely avoid.

Don't move too fast. Keep in mind that heat training takes patience and constantly remind yourself about this fact during your heat training journey. When I first started heat training my hair, I wanted my curls to loosen and I wanted them to loosen fast. I was using my blow dryer and flat iron weekly for the first few months which wasn't the actual problem. The problem was the fact that I wanted fast results and wasn't exercising the patience that was required for this journey. I used a titanium iron (at 450 degrees F) weekly for the first 2 months. My curl pattern loosened extremely fast and fortunately, I didn't experience excessive breakage. I didn't experience a major hair setback because I knew how much heat my hair could tolerate based on my past experience with the use of heat. I also protected my hair with henna, keratin, silicones and with the use of weekly deep steaming treatments. I would not recommend that anyone move this fast on their heat training journey because it is just too risky. In retrospect, I know that I should have moved a lot slower and I shouldn't have been so risky with my hair. It could have turned out awfully bad and I could have easily experienced a hair setback. Although my hair is still thriving, I believe that my hair would have benefitted even more if I had done a slower curl pattern release. I could have used my titanium iron every 2 weeks or even my ceramic iron weekly. I also could have used a titanium iron weekly on a much lower setting. Hindsight is always 20/20.

Heat Training FAQ

I get a lot of questions concerning heat training. Here are some frequently asked questions that I have received.

- **Will heat training my hair make my hair grow?** Not at all. Heat training does not prevent or encourage hair growth. Your hair will continuously grow from your scalp. Whether you heat train (or not) will not affect hair growth at all. The proper use of heat can encourage length retention because your hair will be in its stretched state most of the time. Hair in its stretched state will tend to retain more length due to fewer single strand knots and less tangling/matting.

- **What time of the year is it best to start my heat training journey?**
Although you can start your heat journey at any time of the year, the best time to start is during the fall or winter months AKA "silk press season". This is because during these months, you will be slowly loosening your curl pattern and there is less humidity during this time of year. While you are wearing your hair straight in the fall and winter, it will less likely revert much. As the months pass and you head into the spring and summer, your curl pattern will be much looser and more humidity resistant. You will be able to wear your heat trained

hair in the summer heat with very little reversion.

- **How long will it take for me to heat train my hair?** This answer is different for everyone. It depends on the frequency of your heat training sessions and the temperature settings of your tools. If you are using high heat weekly (in the form of a blow dryer and flat iron), your curls will loosen a lot faster when compared to someone who uses only a blow dryer once per month. It also depends on the degree to which you want your curl pattern loosened. Just a slight break in the disulfide bonds will loosen the curl just a bit and if this is your desired goal, it will happen fairly quickly. I always recommend that you move at a slower pace on your journey so that you can keep a closer eye on the changes occurring with your hair. Using heat every 2 weeks is a great "middle of the road" frequency. You will notice changes in your hair after the 2-month mark. Your hair will be a lot softer and easier to manipulate.

- **Can I use protective styles while heat training?** Certainly! This is a great option for those who need to start their heat training journey in the summer. Protective styling will help to combat serious reversion issues in the humidity. I actually started my heat training journey at the end of the summer and my hair was on the shorter side (about 3 inches). At the beginning of my journey, my hair was reverting very quickly and it was difficult to style because it was so short. My hair was giving James Brown or the Supremes at that time. I maintained my heat training schedule of using heat on my hair every week and I opted for protective styles in between sessions. I would use heat and then put my hair in cornrows. After my cornrows began to frizz, I would wear a curly wig on top of it. I stayed on this regimen until my hair was long enough to wear without protective styling. After a few months, my hair was significantly longer and it wasn't reverting much in the heat.

- **Should I heat train my hair myself or should I go to the salon?** As you have read in this book, heat training is not very difficult to do. If you know how to use a blow dryer and a flat iron, you can definitely heat train your own hair. It may take some practice but after a little repetition, you will be flat ironing your hair with ease. If you still don't feel comfortable heat training your own hair after reading this book, I would suggest that you set up regular appointments with a knowledgeable professional stylist for silk press sessions. Be sure that you and your stylist are on the same page when it comes to loosening your curl pattern and your heat training goals. Communication with your stylist is very important. Be sure to discuss your goals, styling tools, products and home care maintenance.

- **Do I absolutely have to use henna or bond rebuilders while heat training?** Although it is not absolutely necessary, I would suggest that you incorporate one of the two in your hair regimen to strengthen your strands. Bond rebuilders help to partially rebuild the di-sulfide bonds in each strand. This will provide strength and increased elasticity to your hair. They are fairly expensive so be prepared to set money aside in your budget if you go the bond rebuilder route. As mentioned previously, I advocate for the use of henna because it is 100% natural, non-toxic and permanently strengthens and seals the cuticle layer of the hair. It is also extremely inexpensive. Both do a great job at strengthening your hair while heat training.

- **Is steaming really necessary? Can I just deep condition with a heating cap while heat training?** Although steaming is not an absolute necessity, I would definitely recommend this process while on your heat training journey. I have done silk presses with and without the use of steaming. I have to say that it makes a HUGE difference in the final silk press result. Because steaming does a better job at hydrating the hair, the elasticity of the hair is maintained (or may even increase) due to the steaming process. Maintaining your hair's elasticity is very important while heat training. Maintaining optimal moisture in your hair during the deep conditioning process is also equally as important.

- **Can I heat train with only a blow dryer?** Absolutely! Using a blow dryer to heat train will loosen your curl pattern and soften your hair at a much slower rate. It is a great option for those who want to move much slower on their heat training journey and for those

who are just testing the
waters. Using only a blow dryer
is a great way to start if you
have a little anxiety about the
whole notion of heat training.
You will also be able to analyze
how your hair responds to heat
in a more thorough way
because you are progressing
much slower on your journey.

- **What are the best ingredients
  to look for in products while
  heat training my hair?** There
  are 2 very important
  ingredients to look for. Silicone
  (cones) and keratin. These two
  ingredients will be your best
  friends while on your heat
  training journey. Just a few
  years ago, many people
  demonized the use of silicone.
  I'm not exactly sure why. There

were some social media influencers who started bad-mouthing cones and many people followed suit without actually studying the science behind how silicones truly work. Many believed that cones will build up on their hair shaft causing moisture not to be able to enter. This is so far from the truth. Silicones are easily washed out of your hair while deep cleansing. Regular deep cleansing is absolutely essential while on your heat training journey because your hair needs to be in its cleanest state while using heat. This will keep the hair from burning. Because of consistent deep cleansing, silicone will not cause build-up on your hair. Silicone is the absolute best ingredient to protect your hair from burning. In my opinion, silicone is a necessity.

As far as keratin goes, your hair is made of it. It makes up the natural structure of your hair and it is vitally important when it comes to maintaining strong and healthy hair while using heat. This is because it helps to smooth the cuticle. The cuticle layers of the hair actually absorb the keratin once applied (and used with heat) because it is a smaller protein and is compatible with all hair types. In essence, it acts as a protective layer around the hair strand. It guards against the humidity and makes each hair strand reflect light. This gives the hair a brilliant shine.

- **Can I heat train my hair and keep my curls?** Sure! The purpose of heat training is to loosen the bonds of your hair a bit but you can still keep your curls (although they may be slightly loosened). Once you reach the curl pattern that you are comfortable with, lower your heat setting or use heat less frequently to preserve your curls. To maintain your curls after reaching your desired curl pattern, I would suggest using a temperature setting of no more than 400 degrees F and using heat no more than one to two times per month.

- **What if I want my curls back after already loosening them with heat?** Unfortunately, once your curl pattern is loosened with heat, there is not much that you can do to get your hair back to its original state (before heat training). Sometimes the use of bond rebuilders or heavy protein treatment may be able to bring a bit of your curl pattern back but will not bring your hair back to its original 100% natural curl pattern. If you want your natural (virgin) curls back, you will have to cut off your heat trained hair and grow your natural (virgin) hair back. Once the bonds are loosened, it is pretty much permanent.

- **Will I be able to color my hair if I am heat training?** This answer is a bit complex. It really depends on multiple factors. If you are coloring your hair reddish using all-natural henna….. absolutely. Going darker to brown or black with henna and indigo mixtures? Yes! You can definitely get away with using a temporary hair rinse or even a deposit-only color with 5 volume developer (going darker).

If you are interested in lightening your hair with traditional hair color, I would exercise extreme caution because the integrity of each hair strand will be compromised. Lightening your heat trained hair can definitely exacerbate damage because the cortex and cuticle layers of your hair are already compromised and the use of hair color can easily cause irreversible damage. This can result in dry, burned, brittle hair with extreme breakage. Also, if you are heat training your hair, using bleach is certainly not recommended. If you are interested in lightening your hair on your heat training journey, I suggest that you consult a professional who specializes in coloring "natural hair" and obtain recommendations from them.

*Another important point to add is that if you are using henna on your heat training journey and you would like to lighten your hair with traditional hair colors, be very careful. I would seek a professional colorist for these services because mixing henna with traditional colors can cause hair damage with some individuals (if done incorrectly). Remember that henna is permanent and cannot be removed from the hair shaft. You may color your hair darker (deposit color) while using henna with the use of all-natural indigo powder but it is very difficult to lift henna from your hair with commercial hair dyes without experiencing some form of damage. Just keep this in mind.

- **Can I heat train my hair if I am transitioning out of a relaxer?** Absolutely, you can. Just be sure to schedule regular haircuts to get rid of your processed ends. Eventually, your relaxed ends will be gone.

- **Can I just use oil as a heat protectant?** No. This is definitely not a good idea. Contrary to popular belief, oil should not be used as a heat protectant. Oil will heat up on your hair extremely fast and can cause burning of the hair. I suggest that you stick with silicone and keratin-based products to protect your hair from heat.

- **So, are you saying that I shouldn't use oil at all in my hair if I am heat training?** You can definitely use oil in your hair. I just don't suggest using oil in your hair right before using heating tools because the hair can quickly burn. After using your heat tools, feel free to use oil. I don't suggest using too much oil during the first week of your silk press because it will weigh the hair down and it is just not necessary. You can use serums or gloss sprays instead for shine. During week two or three, you can always adjust your regimen as you get closer to your washday. During this time, you can incorporate more lotions and oils as necessary to add moisture and to seal your hair.

- **Why is heat trained hair resistant to humidity?** If you are just starting your heat training journey (on 100% natural/virgin hair), you will notice that your silk press may not last long in any type of humidity. This is because the di-sulfide bonds in your natural hair are super tight and intact. The bonds have not been loosened so any humidity will cause the hair to shrink back up to where it feels comfortable. As you begin to use heat regularly and the bonds are loosened, this will result in a loosened curl pattern. Your hair will be less likely to draw up in the humidity as it did previously. When heat training in conjunction with the use of henna, keratin and silicone-based products, humidity resistance will be even more enhanced. As your heat training journey progresses, your hair's porosity will increase and the keratin and silicone-based products will be able to easily adhere to the cortex layer of your hair strand to fill in the porous gaps. This makes each strand less reactive to humidity. Your hair will not "suck up" the moisture in the air because it is coated properly. Also, I mentioned previously that the use of henna will help your hair resist humidity a great deal because the henna particles bind to the porous gaps along the hair strand causing less humidity to enter. Henna actually helps to prevent reversion.

- **How do I know if my hair is severely damaged from heat?** You will definitely know. There will not be a question. Healthy heat trained natural hair is bouncy, shiny and contains elasticity. Damaged hair will exhibit thinning, breakage, dryness, stiffness, dullness, split ends and a lack of elasticity. If your hair is experiencing any of these forms of damage, I suggest that you start with a fresh haircut and follow the tips in this book to get your heat trained hair healthy. This way, you will retain length and thickness. Holding on to damaged hair will eventually lead to more damage and no progress.

- **Can I change my regimen in the middle of my heat training journey?** Certainly! You can go from only blow drying your hair to blow drying and using a flat iron (and vice versa). You can also adjust your temperature settings and the frequency of heat usage at any time. Be flexible during your heat training journey because your regimen doesn't have to be set in stone. You can change your heat training regimen at any time based on your needs and desired outcome.

- **How do I heat train my hair without causing breakage/ damage?** The key is to follow the tips in this book and "TAKE YOUR TIME". Heat training is a journey and will not happen overnight. In a few months, you will begin to see positive changes in your hair so be patient during the process. Moving too fast during your heat training journey is not advised for the best results.

- **What products should I use daily on my hair after I flat iron it?** This will vary based on the needs of your hair and your desired look. As mentioned previously, I suggest that you not overload your hair with too many products during the flat ironing process and after. This is because too many products will eliminate bounce and body in your hair. A few days after flat ironing your hair, minimal product should be applied to maintain your hair's bounce and flow. As the days pass leading to your wash day, you can add a bit more products to moisturize and seal in the moisture. I am currently on an every 2-week wash schedule. During the first 4-5 days, I use minimal products (if any). On day 5-ish leading up to my wash day, I moisturize with the Hydratherma Naturals Daily Moisturizing Growth Lotion and seal in the moisture with the Hydratherma Naturals Hair Growth Oil every few days. I only use a pea-sized amount or less of each product before wrapping my hair at night. If I feel the need to add a touch of protein, I'll add a pea-sized amount of the Hydratherma Naturals Protein Balance Leave-In Conditioner. These products don't weigh my hair down and keep my hair balanced with moisture and protein during the week.

- **What about touchups during the week with my flat iron if my hair frizzes up a bit?** I unquestionably do not recommend touching up any frizzy areas of your hair with a flat iron after wash day. I know that this seems to be a bit rigid but you do not want to use heat on your hair without it being freshly cleansed. Dust, dirt from the environment, natural oils from the scalp and any residue left from hair products will actually bake into the hair strand. This will eventually cause severe damage in the form of dryness and breakage. When your hair starts to frizz a bit, opt to wear styles with more body. Braid-outs, buns, pin curl sets or any type of curly styles like bantu knot outs …etc. PLEASE. NO DAILY TOUCHIUPS LOL. This will cause a major setback while on your journey.

- **I wear my hair straight all of the time. How can I tell if I am overdoing it with heat?** If your hair has lost its curl pattern, this does not mean that it is burned / severely damaged and requires cutting. Does your hair still feel soft? Is it shiny, healthy looking and strong? If so, you probably are not overusing heat. The signs of true hair damage usually involve dryness, severe split ends, breakage, stiffness, loss of elasticity and dullness. If you notice any of these negative changes in your hair, you are probably overusing heat.

- **Are ponytails really that damaging after silk pressing my hair? Should I avoid them?** You do not have to avoid ponytails altogether. I personally love to wear my hair in a ponytail, especially while I am working out. The key to preventing breakage while wearing a ponytail is to be sure that your ponytail is not too tight, alternate where your ponytail is located and never sleep in your ponytail. Don't wear a bun in your hair while it is wet because this can cause extreme breakage due to the stress on the hair while in its weakened wet state. Another tip is to regularly moisturize and seal in the moisture at the base of where you wear your ponytail the most. Most times, this area of the hair is neglected. One last tip to avoid breakage while wearing ponytails is to never wear ponytail holders with metal on them. One great option is the spiral hair tie. These are like "telephone cord" ponytail holders. I love them because they don't form creases in your hair and they don't pull on the hair at all. This results in less stress and breakage.

-   **This may seem like a silly question but do I have to worry about sun damage, environmental pollution or hard water while I am heat training my hair?** This is definitely not a silly question at all. Yes, these issues are a concern but there are easy remedies that you can incorporate into your hair regimen to prevent your hair from experiencing damage. This is a great question because many people don't think too much about damage occurring from UV rays as well as how air pollution in general can affect the hair in a negative way. Minerals in hard water such as calcium and magnesium can build up on the hair producing a film that makes moisture difficult to penetrate. Chlorine from swimming can have the same effect. UV rays, air pollution and mineral deposits can all cause heat trained hair to become brittle and dry because it is more porous. To prevent this from happening, be sure to protect your hair from sun damage and air pollution with the use of silicone-based products (treatments/leave-in conditioners/serums/heat protectors). Silicones will help to shield your hair and will prevent your hair from experiencing damage from the sun. To remove mineral deposits from your hair, be sure to include clarifying shampoos in your routine. You can also incorporate a chelating shampoo or a baking soda/ apple cider vinegar mixture into your regime (a few times a year) to remove mineral deposits. You can also install a high-quality shower head containing a hard water filter to keep your water "soft". In the end, just a few minor changes can make a big difference when it comes to keeping your hair moisturized, breakage free and healthy.

- **I hate using oils on my hair. My scalp doesn't like it. What can I do?** While wearing a silk press it is not necessary to add oils to your scalp. Your scalp will produce its own natural sebum. I would suggest that you perform scalp massages and brush your hair daily to increase sebum production and encourage growth. The brushing will distribute your natural sebum down the hair strand. As the week progresses (after your wash day), you will notice that your hair will get more naturally oily and this is perfectly normal. The ends of your hair will absolutely love the natural oils that your scalp produces.

- **I have been heat training for 8 months and my hair is now at my bra strap. My hair has never been this long. It isn't breaking or anything and I wear my hair straight all of the time. I keep up with my trims too. I'm just concerned because the ends of my hair are straight and the roots are curly. Should I cut off my straight pieces and start over? I really don't want to cut my hair off.** I get questions like this a lot. You do not have to cut your hair since you are wearing your hair straight all of the time. With heat trained hair, it is absolutely normal for the oldest hair (hair ends) to be straighter than the roots. Your hair ends have been exposed to more heat so the curl pattern will be looser of course. The newest hair (closer to the root) will be curlier because it hasn't been exposed to as much heat. It sounds like your hair is in great shape because you are not experiencing breakage and you are keeping up with your trims. Plus, you mentioned that you are retaining length and that you wear your hair straight all of the time. I don't think that you should worry about your straight ends and I definitely don't suggest that you cut them off. This is all part of the heat training journey. Some people heat train their hair until there is almost no curl pattern left and some people still have some curl definition. My hair ends are 80% straight when it is wet and my hair is thriving. There is no need to cut your hair. Just continue on your heat training journey and continue to use the tips/ regimens in this book to maintain your healthy hair.

- **Saleemah, what exactly is your current hair regimen now that your hair is already heat trained?** My hair is super easy to maintain at this point. My hair is currently heat trained to the level that I am very comfortable with. Since my hair ends are no longer needing to be "trained", I primarily focus on my hair roots as they grow out. I apply more heat to my roots and only use one pass of the flat iron on my hair ends. I am using the Hydratherma Naturals Silk Press System and use heat on my hair approximately every 2 weeks in the form of a blow dryer and flat iron. I do incorporate steaming with each wash day session for about 10 minutes.

I use my blow dryer on high and I keep the temperature of my flat iron at around 430 degrees F for a silky straight look. If I don't want a bone straight look, I will use lower heat settings like 370-400 degrees F. I wrap my hair at night and use minimal products for the first week. During the second week, I usually incorporate oils and/or moisturizers to my hair regimen with products such as the Hydratherma Naurals Protein Balance Leave In Conditioner, Daily Moisturizing Growth Lotion and the Hair Growth Oil. These products help to balance the moisture and protein levels in my hair to prevent breakage. I use only a pea sized amount on my hair before wrapping so that my hair is not weighed down.

If I want to add curls to my hair during the week, I don't reapply heat because this can be extremely damaging. I just utilize pin-curls, head band curls, sock curls or bantu knots to set my hair before bed. I typically use the Hydratherma Naturals Foaming Sea Silk Curly Styler for long lasting curls the next day.

When I go to the gym, I regularly wear my hair in 2 high ponytails. I like to wear 2 ponytails instead of one because when I sweat, the middle section of my hair can dry faster. After my work-out is done, I let my hair air dry in the ponytails. If you are in a rush, you can use a cool hair dryer. Once dry, I wrap my hair and let it set. When I take my wrap down, my hair looks flawless.

The ends of my hair are pretty straight when wet. This is the level of heat training that I desired and this is not necessary for everyone. As I mentioned previously, you can heat train your hair and keep some of your curl pattern if you wish. It just depends on your comfort level. It also depends on how your hair reacts to heat as you monitor it during your heat training journey. This is why closely monitoring your hair is very significant.

At this point on my heat training journey, when I blow dry my hair, the results are pretty straight without using a flat iron. I can just blow dry my hair and flat iron the roots if I don't want a silky straight look.

Hair Product Recommendations

Styling Tools / Henna Brand Recommendations- These are all of the heat-styling tools that I truly believe in. All of the heat styling tools and henna products that I recommend are not sponsored recommendations. I am not being paid to promote them. These are the henna products and styling tools that I personally love and use on a regular basis.

Tools

Kipozi Brand- V7 Titanium Flat Iron- The Kipozi brand is very affordable averaging $30.00 and up. I have to say that these are some of the best titanium flat irons that I have ever used. I have used many other bands costing 10X the price and these irons work just as well or even better. I have heard that this company is rebranding and changing its name in the near future, so keep that in mind if you are looking to purchase this iron.

FHI Platform Ceramic Iron- If you want to go the ceramic route, I would suggest this FHI flat iron. It runs about $120.00. Smooths the hair easily and effortlessly. It is very lightweight and easy to use.

FHI Platform Handle-less Hair Dryer- This is one of my favorite blow dryers because it is handle-less. It is super easy to grip and control. It also provides ceramic heat and negative ions which cuts my blowout time in half. It comes with its own comb attachment which contributes to a smoother / straighter blowout. It takes me about 10 minutes to thoroughly blow-dry all of my hair.

Henna

Godrej Nupur Henna- This brand is a 100% pure henna product and the only brand of henna that I trust. It only contains Lawsonia inermis leaf powder (mehendi) as the listed ingredient. There is also a Nupur "9 herb" version which contains additional herbs including Shikakai, Aloe Vera, Methi, Hibiscus, Jatamansi, Bhringraj, Amla, Neem, Brahmi. Both visions are 100% pure and don't contain any metallic salts. As I mentioned previously, many products that are labeled as "henna" are not pure and may contain many damaging chemicals.

Silk Press Product Recommendations

I am recommending Hydratherma Naturals products for heat training natural hair not only because I own the brand but because I wholeheartedly stand behind our products 100%. I truly believe that our products are among of the highest quality products in the market. All of the below products are part of the Hydratherma Naturals Silk Press System which is currently available at www.HydrathermaNaturals.com, www.HealthyHairJourney.com, Amazon and at retail locations listed on our website.

As mentioned previously, there are certain qualities and ingredients that make up amazing silk press products. If you want your hair to be shiny, bouncy and protected from burning, give the below products a try while on your heat training journey.

Step 1: Shampoo

Deep cleanse your hair with the Hydratherma Naturals cleansers. Be sure to remove all excess dirt and buildup. This is very important. The perfect silk press starts will properly cleansed hair.

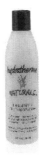

Hydratherma Naturals Herbal Amino Clarifying Shampoo (Lather 1)

☐ Removes Buildup & Residue Without Stripping Your Hair of Natural Oils

☐ Enriched with Keratin Amino Acids to Strengthen Your Hair

☐ Enhanced with Multiple Botanicals Including Lemongrass, Kiwi Fruit and Quercus Alba Bark Extracts

☐ Hydrating

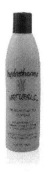

Hydratherma Naturals Moisture Boosting Shampoo (Lather 2)

☐ Contains Multiple Natural Extracts Including Seaweed, Algae & Sea Kelp

☐ Delivers Omega 3 And Omega 6 Essential Acids to Each Hair Strand

☐ Moisturizes the Scalp, Reduce Dryness, Decreases Dandruff & Regulates Sebaceous Secretion.

☐ Offers Extreme Hydration

☐ Concentrated Formula. A little Goes a Very Long Way

Step 2: Deep Conditioning Treatment

Section your hair into 4 sections and apply the Peppermint Cream Ultimate Nourishing Deep Conditioner from root to tip, comb through (removing all tangles) and proceed to steam your hair for 10-20 minutes. Rinse. Allow the last 10 seconds to be a cold rinse to close your cuticle.

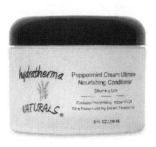

Hydratherma Naturals Peppermint Cream Ultimate Nourishing Deep Conditioner

☐ Adds Layers of Protection to the Hair Prior to Using Heat.

☐ Restore Moisture and Protein Balance to Silk Pressed / Heat Treated Hair

☐ Prevents Breakage with Rice Protein to Strengthen Hair Fibers

☐ Contains Ivy Root Extract to Control Greasy / Itchy Scalp

☐ Stimulates Scalp and Encourages Growth with Fenugreek Seed,

Burdock Root and Peppermint Oil Extracts

Step 3: Leave-In Conditioning Treatment

Re-section your hair into 4 sections. Apply the Chia Seed Moisture Fix Leave-In Conditioner to prevent breakage, detangle, increase shine, hydrate and provide heat protection. Only a pea size amount is needed per section for adequate protection. Do not overuse.

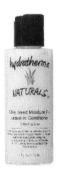

Hydratherma Naturals Chia Seed Moisture Fix Leave In Conditioner

☐ Contains a Unique Infusion of Chia Seed & Henna Extracts to Coat and Protect Each Strand from Heat

☐ Restores Elasticity and Adds Moisture / Protein Balance to Heat Treated Hair

☐ Recovers Maximum Moisture and Protection Prior to Using Heat.

☐ Amazing Detangler- Detangles Your Hair from Root to Tip

☐ Contains Vegetable Proteins to Strengthen Each Strand

☐ Resist Hair Breakage and Promotes Healthy Heat-Treated Hair

☐ Contains Silicones for Optimal Heat Protection and Humidity Resistance

Step 4: Serum

To all 4 sections, apply a pea size
amount of the Keratin Glass
Advanced Smoothing Serum to
smooth, provide humidity resistance,
seal the cuticle, strengthen and add a
brilliant shine. Brush each section
with your detangling brush to evenly
distribute the products. There is no
need to overuse this product. The
Keratin Glass will allow the flat iron to
easily glide through the hair without
causing snags. After using this
product, proceed to blow dry.

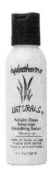

Hydratherma Naturals Keratin Glass Advanced Smoothing Serum

☐ Enriched with Keratin Protein & Algae Extracts to Coat and Protect Each Strand from Heat

☐ Provides Humidity Resistance to Heat Treated Hair

☐ Seals the Cuticle and Controls Frizz

☐ Detangles Your Hair from Root to Tip and allows the flat iron to easily glide through the hair without causing snags.

☐ When used with Heat, Brilliant Shine and Smoothing are Intensified

☐ Lightweight and will not Weight Your Hair Down.

☐ Promotes Healthy Heat-Treated Hair by Adding a Layer of Protection

☐ Contains Silicone for Optimal Heat Protection and Humidity Resistance

Step 5: Gloss

Finally, apply only 2-3 uniform strokes of the Herbal Gloss Heat Protector (to your entire head of blow-dried hair) for additional heat protection and a brilliant shine. Hold bottle 10-12 inches from hair. Proceed to flat iron your hair.

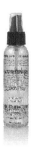

Herbal Gloss Heat Protector

☐ Softens- Conditions- Adds Extreme Shine

☐ Protects Your Hair from Irreversible Heat Damage

☐ Contains Protective Filters to Help Prevent Heat / Sun Damage.

☐ Herbal Formula to Strengthen Your Hair

☐ Can be used Daily to Add Shine to Any Style

*For a smooth press from root to tip, I recommend the **Hydratherma Naturals Flat Iron Chase Comb** to prevent frizzy ends. This comb is more effective when compared to a rat tail comb because it actually grips the hair.

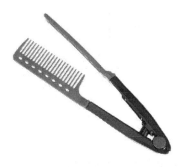

This innovative styling comb controls even sections of hair allowing you to more effectively apply heat from your dryer or flat iron. Holds hair taut to help reach every hair strand for smoother / straighter ends. It is designed with a hinged handle that is spring-loaded to open when released. When closed the two ends of the comb meet (as the teeth slide into holes in the opposing end) closing tight. This will allow you to "lock" the section of the hair and apply the necessary tension.

Conclusion

I'm sure that you purchased this book because you felt the need to alter your hair care regimen and create an easier routine that works well for your lifestyle (without the use of chemicals). Now that you have completed this book, I hope that you have gained all of the information that you need to make an informed decision about heat training your hair. If you do decide to embark on this journey, you now have the knowledge to heat train your hair correctly and with confidence. You can now sit down and create an action plan.

Heat training is a very controversial topic to some

individuals but it works for many. I'm sure that the information in this book has confirmed to be very helpful for those looking for a chemical-free option. I am so happy that I embarked on my heat training journey and I'm sure that you will too. Be confident with your decision and do what works well for you and your hair.

Cheers to healthy heat trained hair!!!

About the Author

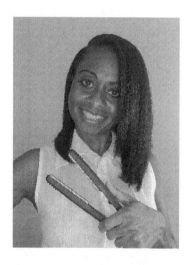

An entrepreneur, author, licensed cosmetologist and registered nurse (BSN). Saleemah Cartwright, founder and co-owner of the Hydratherma Naturals healthy hair care product collection, has made it her mission to promote healthy hair by developing superior hair care products & systems that benefit consumers and support the environment.

Committed to inspiring, educating and empowering consumers about achieving healthy hair, she encourages her customers to reach their goals through healthy hair care practices. She is also the co-founder of Healthy Hair Journey Enterprises L.L.C.

"Hair is my love! Hair is my passion! To see hair flourish, thrive and prosper gives me excitement. I find my passion through helping others reach their healthy hair goals. I thank God for the opportunity to share my love with others!" -Saleemah Cartwright

Additional Resource

Book
"300 Healthy Hair Tips for All Hair Types"

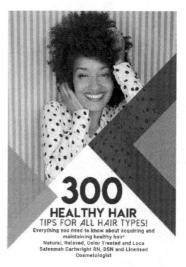

If you would like to dive a lot deeper into general healthy hair care practices for all hair types, please take a look at my 1st book titled, "300 Healthy Hair Tips for all Hair Types". This book will give you 300

simple tips, techniques and secrets to help you reach your healthy hair goals. Includes tips for natural hair, relaxed hair, color-treated hair and locs. Available at HydrathermaNaturals.com and Amazon.

Follow us on social media to learn more about heat training.

HealthyHairJourney.com or
HydrathermaNaturals.com

Facebook.com/Hydratherma

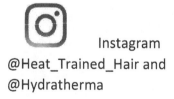 Instagram
@Heat_Trained_Hair and
@Hydratherma

Twitter / X @Hydratherma

 TikTok
@Heat_Trained_Hair and
@Hydratherma

 YouTube/ Saleemah
Cartwright

 Pinterest
@HydrathermaPins

HealthyHairJourney@yahoo.com

Disclaimer

Every effort has been made to ensure the accuracy of the information/material contained in this book. The authentic contents in this book are written and researched to the best of the author's knowledge and as such cannot be guaranteed free of error or with the absence of key information.
The information in this book is intended to provide general information regarding hair care practices and product suggestions. It is not to be construed as medical/professional advice or instruction. All information in

specific to your situation. All information and resources found in this book are based on the opinions of the author, unless otherwise noted. We accept no liability for any claim, for loss or damage arising from the use of this book or product recommendations made. Our solutions, instructions, and recommendations are to be followed at your own risk and discretion and we are not to be held liable. The products recommended are what have been found to work for many, but they may not provide the same results for all individuals. Each individual is different. Certain products and procedures or solutions may potentially cause an intolerance, allergy, or hair damage/hair loss therefore the author explicitly states that the use of any products, methods, solutions, or recommendations found in this book is at your own risk and discretion and we are not to be held liable. Prior to using the products recommended in this book, please first read the information/ instructions on the packaging label.

---

written permission of the
copyright holder.

Made in the USA
Columbia, SC
26 February 2024

32013910R00135